CW01017850

PREFACE

The literature in orthopaedics is immense; there is a book of 500 pages devoted to the front half of the foot!

I have written this book as a guide to better understanding of the subject.

I have been greatly influenced by the late Alan Graham Apley who believed in simple English, was a superb teacher, a fine orthopaedic surgeon and author of a comprehensive textbook on Orthopaedics, which is recommended for further reading.

I dedicate this book to his memory.

I can also recommend "The Story of Orthopaedics" by Mercer Rang.

Acknowledgements

My thanks are due to Jackie Chippette for help with the typing and formerly to Jo & Joe Design for help with previous editions. I acknowledge the authors of the cartoons used. My thanks also to the staff at Trident Printing for their help.

CONTENTS

FOREWORD

We communicate by words and the meaning can be misinterpreted when one person says something and the other person hears something else or misconstrues what is meant.

This is particularly true when a consultation takes place between a doctor and a patient, especially if a word the doctor uses is Latinised. A person can believe a fracture is worse than a break when they both mean the same.

Sometimes a word is emotive like cancer or whiplash, and when one hears the word cancer one fears death will follow when it may be a benign or harmless growth.

The internet does not always provide the best source of knowledge but is enormously helpful is finding out about certain conditions.

The history of medicine is full of examples when an idea is not acceptable because it is new and runs contrary to what is believed. William Harvey found the circulation of the blood in 1625 but his colleagues had been taught from Galen's time (1500 years before) that the heart pumped the blood back and forth like the tides going in and out and would not accept the new concept that blood was pumped around the body and back again. It seems laughable now, but not then.

An idea such as washing one's hands to prevent carrying infection from one person to another took over a hundred years before it was accepted and even then the discovery of the microscopic organisms did not convince everyone.

Nicholas Andry, Professor of Medicine in Paris in 1741, devised the word *"Orthopaedia"* as a title for a book he wrote on the methods of preventing deformities in children. He devised the word from two Greek words *orthos* meaning straight and *pais* meaning child or *paedia* the study of children. The tree on the cover of this book is meant to donate that the spine of the child with splintage will grow straight as will the tree.

This tree has become the symbol of every Orthopaedic Society throughout the English-speaking world.

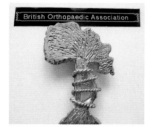

This is the lapel badge of the British Orthopaedic Asociation.

Orthopaedics itself has grown to include adults as well as children and is concerned with the musculoskeletal system.

WHERE WE COME FROM

It all started with the big bang about 13.5 billion years ago, when the Universe was born and formed huge numbers of subatomic particles which condensed to form huge numbers of the basic atom of hydrogen. This has a single nucleus with a proton (positively charged) and neutron (no charge) surrounded by an electron (negatively charged) and these were blasted into space and are still expanding.

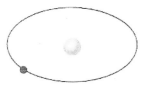

Hydrogen Atom

Clumps of hydrogen atoms condensed to form stars and the internal pressure was such that two atoms of hydrogen were fused to form helium giving off immense energy in the form of heat and light. When a star grew too big or two stars collided a supernova explosion fused atoms together to form the remaining elements of the periodic table.

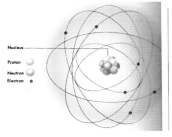

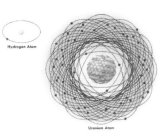

Carbon (6 protons and 6 electrons)   Uranium (92 protons and electrons)

These were blasted into space and condensed to form planets and became trapped by the gravitational pull of a nearby star.

Our solar system was born about 4 billion years ago.

The earth was very hot and grew with the impact of various meteors and comets containing water.

Eventually cooling allowed the oceans to form and a water cycle with evaporation to form clouds and rain commenced.

Life developed in the primordial oceans about 3 billion years ago by combining proteins called amino acids.

A coiled molecule of DNA (deoxyribonucleic acid) formed which was capable of splitting and living organisms developed.

This process continued as evolution and eventually humans arrived about 3 million years ago, with modern man about 20000 years ago. If you condense the history of the planet of 4 billion years to 24 hours humans have been around for the last 5 seconds.

Early humans looked like this, and their paintings are recorded in the caves of the Perigord in France, in Spain and Australia:

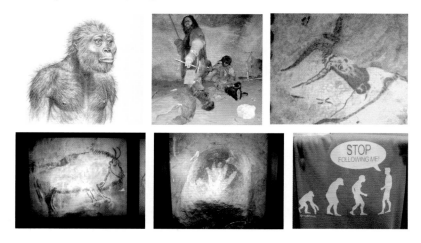

This was from a T shirt showing the ascent of man from early humanids

WHAT WE ARE MADE OF

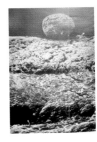 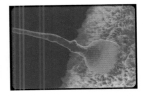 When a sperm and an egg unite they form a new organism which starts to divide. Note the size of the sperm at the bottom of the left picture as it approaches the egg. The cells divide and reproduce and within three to four days the multinucleated cell implants into the wall of the uterus and continues to grow. Stem cells divide into three basic tissues. Up to eight weeks the developing baby is called an embryo and after that a foetus.

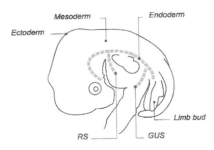

6 Week old Embryo

Ectoderm   which gives rise to the nervous system and the skin.

Endoderm   which gives rise to the alimentary canal, its lining and the glandular structures that develop from it such as the liver and pancreas; also the respiratory and genitourinary system

Mesoderm   which gives rise to the muscles, bones and joints or the musculoskeletal system.

Nutrition from the mother develops via a placenta and after eight weeks the

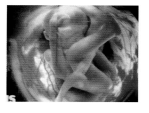

embryo becomes a recognisable human foetus and spends the remaining time in the uterus until a viable age (now reduced to 24 weeks) arrives, although most babies need until 40 weeks or nine months before they are sufficiently able to survive the cold, hard world outside the womb.

The body consists of many different sets of **tissues**, made up of **cells** with a similar function, called **systems**. They are all interdependent.

NS - Nervous System where the brain's impulses are received analysed and impulses transmitted to effect the various other organs via the **spinal cord**. Grey matter is the cells (**neurons**) and white matter the strands (**dendrites** or **axons**) which transmit the impulses. The surface is convoluted or folded and if spread out would be the size of a pillowcase. Because the brain analyses thoughts and emotions a subdivision could be called the **psychological system**.

CVS - CardioVascular System is concerned with the heart which pumps oxygenated blood throughout the body and deoxygenated blood returning from the rest of the body, pumped through the lungs for re-oxygenation and back to the heart for circulation through the blood vessels, arteries, capillaries and veins.

RS - Respiratory System consists of passages from the nose and mouth to the lungs where oxygen exchange takes place and gaseous waste products are excreted.

AS - Alimentary System consists of the mouth and gut where food is ingested, digested, absorbed and excreted.

MSS - Musculo-Skeletal System consists of the bones and joints and the muscles that move them.

GUS - Genito-Urinary System consists of the kidneys, tubes and bladder filtering waste products from the blood excreting them in the urine; and the reproductive organs.

LS - Lymphatic System consists of the tiny channels that bring fluids leaked from the blood vessels back into the blood vascular system, via nodes (often, wrongly, called glands) which filter bacteria or neoplastic cells, and can become inflamed and swollen.

HS - Haemo-poietic System concerns the manufacture of red and white blood cells and platelets, in the spleen and bone marrow.

ES - Endocrine System where hormones that control metabolism or various other functions of the body are made.

There are three different types of cells that make up the different systems:

Labile: These are capable of reproduction and usually do reproduce all the time. It is said that the whole skeleton is usually replaced within seven years as old bone is taken away and new bone is laid down (fortunately not all at once). Cells are lost continuously from the skin surface; and from the lining of the gut and lungs. These cells are the ones that usually respond to extraneous stimuli to become malignant.

The suffix –**blast** is used to describe cell formation such as osteoblasts or bone (osteo) forming cells; -**clast** or -**phage** to describe cells that break down tissue (osteoclasts), macrophages blood cells that ingest and break down tissue; and –**cyte** to denote stable cells (osteocyte -bone cells).

Stable: These cells are only capable of reproduction when needed such as cells within the liver.

Permanent: These cells lack the ability to reproduce and damage to these cells is usually permanent. Nerve cells, muscle cells (myocytes), and cells forming the cartilage lining joints (chondrocytes) fall into this category.

MUSCULOSKELTAL SYSTEM

We form part of a group of animals known as vertebrates which have an **endoskeleton** or bones within the body and there are features common to all. There is a central vertebral column and from which arise the rib cage and four **pentadactyl** (five dactyls or digits) limbs. These are modified in different animals such that the upper arms become wings in birds and the toes turned around to be able to grip twigs and branches.

In the human skeleton there are 33 vertebrae supporting a head at one end and articulating with the pelvis at the other with a rib cage, arms on either side and legs.

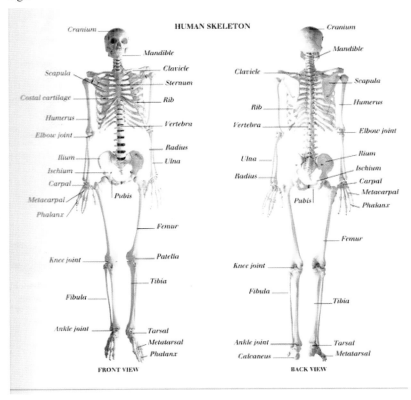

The bones meet at **joints.** There are fixed joints such as where the ribs meet the breast bone (**cartilaginous** joints), semi-fixed joints (**fibrous** joints) such as between the vertebrae or where the pelvic bones meet in the front and mobile joints (**synovial** joints).

A synovial joint is so called because the bone ends are lined by **hyaline cartilage** which needs lubricating by the fluid secreted by the **synovial membrane** lining the capsule of the joint. The capsule is an enclosing membrane which is thickened in some parts by fibrous tissue called **ligaments**, restricting movements in some planes but not in others. The cartilage is sometimes reinforced by a **meniscus** made of fibrocartilage (commonly called cartilages in the knee) which may be partial, as in the knee, or complete as in the temporomandibular (jaw) joint.

Synovial Joint

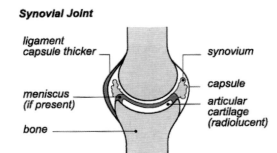

There are various types of joints such as ball and socket joints where free movement is allowed in various directions, hinge joints such as the elbow, combination joints such as the knee where some rotation is allowed and facet joints in the spine. There are pivot joints where the head meets the spinal column at the atlas to allow nodding and swivel joints such as below the atlas with the dens of the axis vertebra to allow turning. There are some joints called saddle joints such as the base of the thumb which allow movement in different directions.

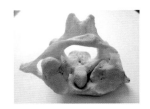

Atlas below, axis above

13

Bones are made of **a fibrous tissue** set in **calcium hydroxyapatite** (similar to chalk). It is the calcium which blocks x-rays producing the shadow on the film first discovered by Roentgen in 1906.

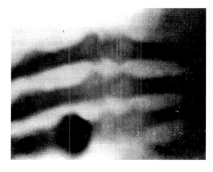

This is Roentgen's original x-ray of his wife's hand with her ring taken after 6 minutes exposure. It created huge interest when he first published his results and over 1000 papers were produced in the year afterwards! Barium salts ingested, were used to display the stomach and intestines.

Long bones are hollow to provide lightness with strength. They are lined with dense fibrous tissue called **periosteum** which has the ability to make bone and is used to provide attachment to the muscles and tendons. The hollow is filled with marrow, which in children is **haemopoietic** producing red and white blood cells. In adults the marrow is replaced by liquid **fat** which in fractures may penetrate the vascular system producing a syndrome called fat embolism.

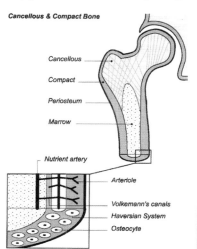

There are two types of bony tissue.

Compact bone: This is dense bone made up of Haversian systems with a lot of hydroxyapatite between the systems producing a dense appearance on x-rays.

Cancellous bone: This is made up of bony **trabeculae** usually aligned in the direction of force applied to the bone and consists of thin plates of bone interspersed with haemopoietic tissue. Bone is similar to a Crunchy bar where the periosteum is the silver wrapping, the chocolate on the outside is the compact bone and the honeycomb is the cancellous bone on the inside.

Bony growth occurs at the ends of long bone at the **epiphysis** which is made up of cartilage cells multiplying, hypertrophying and calcifying and being replaced by bone (**metaphysis**). The **apophysis** is the growth plate on the side of the bone, such as the front of the proximal tibia,or back of the os calcis (heel bone). **Remodelling** occurs to ensure that the bone grows symmetrically. This however is also determined by forces applied to the bone and because of the curled up nature of the foetus in the uterus the baby is born with bent legs which take about 12 months to straighten out. However deficiencies of Vitamin D may also produce bowing of the legs called rickets.

Growth Plate

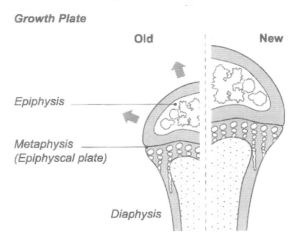

Bony growth ceases at the end of adolescence although the last epiphysis to close is the inner end of the clavicle around the age of 24.

Bone requires a blood supply and is in a constant state of removal and replacement according to the stresses laid upon it. Bone reacts to stress or irritation by either laying down bone due to over activity of the **osteoblasts** which are the cells that form bone and hardening of the bone is described as **osteosclerosis (-sclerosis means hardening)**. Bone is removed by the **osteoclasts** and this produces **osteoporosis** (generalised loss), or **cysts** (localised loss). Stable bone cells are called **osteocytes**. In some circumstances a mixed picture may appear in various disease processes such as Paget's disease where bone can be thickened and bent.

Muscles:

There are various types of muscle fibre such as **cardiac** muscle which is specialised to provide rhythmic contraction continuously throughout life.

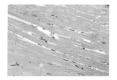

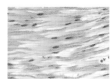

There is **smooth** muscle which is found in the wall of the gut providing peristalsis and the movement of food through the alimentary canal. Smooth muscle is also found in some blood vessels which dilate when we blush and constrict when we see a ghost for example.

The muscles that move the joints are called **striated** muscles because of their

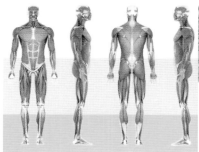

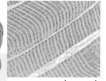

appearance under the microscope. They are formed into bundles that contract in unison in response to nervous stimuli. Energy is released in the cells and working muscles need a rich blood supply. If an accumulation of waste products occurs cramp sets in. They are extended by tendons of bundles of **collagen fibres** (similar to a rope) and form a strong attachment to bone. Tendons slide within a sheath and are lubricated by synovial fluid. If a muscle contacts too violently it can tear the muscle fibres themselves or the tendons.

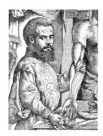

This is a woodcut of Andreas Vesalius whose book "De Humani Corporis Fabricus" published in 1543 showed a detailed dissection of the way the body was made up of its various organs, muscles,vessels and bones. He laid the foundation of observation and research fundamental to all discovery.

WHAT CAN GO WRONG

This is called **pathology**. Sometimes the developing cells do not grow correctly and these conditions are called **congenital**. Often it is based on faulty genes and more and more conditions are now being diagnosed and sometimes corrected in utero. Detailed conditions will be considered later. **Acquired** conditions come on throughout life. Many words in medicine have prefixes or suffixes to clarify their meaning and most are based on Latin or Greek. They affect the different systems in the body.

Inflammation, Inflammatory (-itis)

Acute/chronic: Tissues react to irritation such as from bacteria or chemicals by the production of fluid and the invasion of white cells and macrophages. **Pus** is this fluid and dead bacteria. A collection of pus is called an **abscess.**

The suffix *-itis* is applied to the organ affected such as tonsillitis, appendicitis, osteomyelitis. 2000 years ago the Greek, Celsus, described the following as the effects of inflammation:
Rubor, redness.
Dolor pain.
Calor, heat.
Tumor, swelling, to which maybe added
Loss of function.

My hero in medicine is Ambroise Paré who lived from 1510 to 1590. When he was a young doctor he joined the army as a surgeon and there were various wars being fought in Europe at that time. It is better to let him describe in his own words what happened:

"I had not yet seen gunshot wounds at the first dressing. I had read in Jean De Vigo's book " Of Wounds in General" Chapter 8 that wounds made by firearms partake of venomosity, by reason of the gunpowder, and for their cure he bids you cauterise them with oil of elder, scalding hot, mixed with a little treacle. And to make no mistake, before I would use this said oil, knowing it was to bring great pain to the patient I asked first, before I applied it, what the other surgeons used for the first dressing; which was to put the said oil, boiling well, into the wounds, and tents and setons; wherefore I took courage to do as they did. At last my oil ran short; and I was compelled instead of it, to apply a digestive made of yolk of eggs, oil of roses and turpentine. In the night I could not sleep in quiet, fearing some default in not cauterising, lest I should find those, to whom I had not applied the said oil, dead from the poison of their wounds; which made me rise very early to visit them; where, beyond my expectation, I found that they to whom I had applied my digestive had suffered but little pain in their wounds without inflammation or swelling, having rested fairly well that night. The others to whom the boiling oil was applied, I found feverish, with great pain, and swelling around the edges of their wounds. Then I resolved never more to burn these cruelly poor men with gunshot wounds".

This is a very good description of the inflammatory reaction to boiling oil and also a lesson to not believe everything that one reads in established text books, or is taught.

Trauma, Traumatic: This is injury to a tissue with the result depending 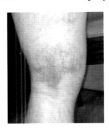 on the force and the tissues to which it is applied. For example, soft tissue may be bruised, or bone broken. Signs of inflammation are present. Bleeding into the tissues produces a **haematoma** (swelling) and colour changes as the blood is broken down e.g. a torn hamstring.

Neoplasia, Neoplastic: *Neo new and **Plasia** growth.* New growth of tissues independent of normal control (**tumour-** which really means swelling). The body does not recognise that they may be harmful and feeds them often causing death in malignant tumours that are not successfully treated.

Benign (-oma): This is a tumour which remains localised to the area. The suffix *-oma* is applied to the tissue such as lipoma (a fatty tumour), fibroma (a fibrous tumour). The effects produced depend on the situation. Swelling may be visible and pain may be produced from pressure on sensitive surrounding tissue.

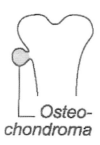

Osteo-
chondroma

Malignant (-carcinoma, -sarcoma):

These tumours invade the surrounding tissue and metastasise or spread to distant parts via lymphatics or the blood stream. These secondary deposits are known as **metastases** or **secondaries**.

Carcinoma: This usually applied to the tissues derived from the ectoderm and endoderm such as squamous cell carcinoma of the skin, adenocarcinoma of the breast, adenocarcinoma of the stomach. Early spread is to the lymph nodes and later via the blood stream.

Sarcoma: This usually applies to tissues derived from the mesoderm such as fibrosarcoma, osteosarcoma or myosarcoma.

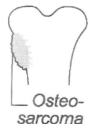

Early spread is via the blood stream. The effects depend on the rate of growth of the tumour and how quickly it spreads.

Superficial tumours are more quickly diagnosed and treatment is often effective before they have spread. Cancer is a word commonly used, but is wrongly used, and creates fear as not all malignant tumours are fatal. The problem is that the body recognises the malignant cell as belonging to it and feeds it.

Degenerative (-osis):

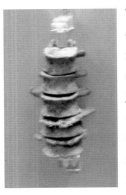

This is ageing of the tissues and occurs to us all. **Spondylosis** means degeneration of the **spine** and **arthrosis** degeneration of a **joint** (arthrus) although by common usage arthritis is the more commonly used term. This spine is from the British Museum Mummy section and shows a 2000 year old spine with marked degenerative changes. I am sure he would have had back ache!! **Sclerosis** means hardening and arterio-sclerosis is hardening of the arteries by deposits of calcium in the walls lining them. **Stenosis** means narrowing and is seen in chronic degeneration in the spine.

Metabolic: This involves the energy and chemical processes in the body such as too much uric acid from the breakdown of amino acids producing gout and crystals in the joint causing pain.

Endocrine: This affects the various glands in the body such as an overactive pituitary producing excess growth in children with gigantism, or, in adults, acromegaly. Diabetes is altered production of insulin moderating blood sugar levels.

Immunological: Disorders of the immune system such as rheumatoid arthritis or AIDS (auto-immune deficiency syndrome).

Pyschosomatic: This is where the person believes there is a problem when there is no organic cause and when carried to excess is commonly called Munchausen's syndrome.

Iatrogenic: This is a medical complication such as injecting a nerve producing damage.

Idiopathic: This is where no cause is found.

HOW TO FIX IT

This depends on establishing a **diagnosis,** or cause of a condition. A diagnosis is based on history, examination and investigation (symptoms, signs, tests). Various conditions are considered and a list of priorities drawn up **(differential diagnosis). Common things occur commonly.**

SYMPTOMS: These are complaints made by the patient and the commonest in musculoskeletal conditions is pain. Different people are affected differently and some people are more stoic than others. Pain is an emotive term and can be superficial or deep. Superficial pain often produces words like burning or scalding, a feeling like ants under the skin or sharp like a pinprick. Deep pain uses words like aching or crushing. Litigation has been shown to prolong symptoms in some cases, possibly due to an unconscious desire to punish the other party. However they do not always resolve when the case is settled. Sometimes patients fall into the **sick role syndrome** where they get attention from other members of the family that they may not have had before. Sometimes symptoms are fabricated as in the Munchausen syndrome and doctors are led on various wild goose chases that may even involve surgery, before it is recognised. In writing up a case history it is usually under different headings such as:

PC   Present complaints.

HPI   History of the present illness.

FH   Family history.

SH   Social history.

SIGNS: These are findings on examination:

General Examination: The doctor usually starts an observation as soon as a patient enters the consulting room and a lot can be learned from the demeanour, facial expression and behaviour. A person can be seen to be in agony by the expression on their face. Chronic pain can cause deep shadows under the eyes and a gaunt expression. When faced with such a person who says there is little wrong with them a doctor must beware. Similarly, a person who describes chronic pain but is not obviously in pain and who has a normal appearance with little to show on their face may be just seeking attention. A lot can be learnt by how the patient describes their condition and their tone of voice.

Local Examination:

Look   inspection – the part may be red and swollen suggesting an infection.

Feel   palpation- gentle pressure may cause acute pain or there may be rebound pain when the hand is lifted suddenly from the abdomen, for example, in appendicitis.

Move   percussion- tapping an area may produce a dull sound or moving a joint may cause pain.

Hear   auscultation- sometimes joints creak when moved or there may be crackles and wheezes heard when listening to the lungs. The stethoscope was invented to protect the modesty of female patients when examining the chest.

The terms used help to understand the location of the problem.

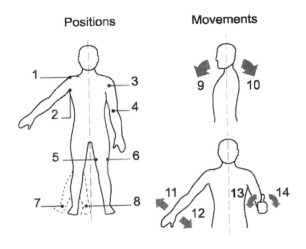

Positions   Movements

Anterior is in front, **posterior** behind and **lateral** to the side.

1.	**Supra-/superior**	Above
2.	**Infra-/inferior**	Below
3.	**Proximal**	Towards the top
4.	**Distal**	Towards the bottom
5.	**Medial**	On the inner side
6.	**Lateral**	On the outer side
7.	**Valgus**	Away from the midline
8.	**Varus**	Towards the midline
9.	**Flexion**	Bending forwards
10.	**Extension**	Bending backwards
11.	**Abduction**	Movement away from the midline
12.	**Adduction**	Movement towards the midline
13.	**Pronation**	Rotating inwards
14.	**Supination**	Rotating outwards

All joints are at $0°$ in the erect position except during pronation and supination where with the elbow flexed at $90°$ and thumb is up is $0°$.

24

***TESTS*:**   If the diagnosis is in doubt or to confirm diagnosis tests are carried out either on an outpatient or inpatient basis. They are expensive and should not be ordered indiscriminately.

X-ray: AP (antero-posterior or front to back)   Lateral (sideways) Oblique views are necessary to obtain the best information.

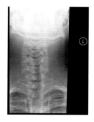

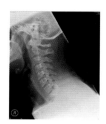

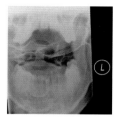

Cervical spine AP   Lateral   Open mouth view as the jaw obscures the uppermost vertebrae

Blood: A full blood screen to include red cell count, white cell count, ESR (erythrocyte sedimentation rate: the rate at which red cells drop in plasma), blood chemistry e.g. raised uric acid in gout. Blood culture if infection is suspected.

Urine: Blood, protein, organisms and crystals.

Sputum: Culture, cytology.

SPECIAL INVESTIGATIONS:

Computerised Axial Tomography (CT): A special x-ray showing sections through the body.

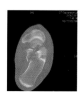 This shows a fracture on the inner side of the calcanuem or heel bone. Here is a CT of the upper Cervical spine showing scatter due to metallic fillings in the teeth.

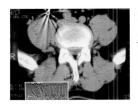

Here is an unusual scatter from a small linear object just visible in front of the vertebrae on the bottom of the picture and is hollow. It was the appendix with barium from a barium enema some days before.

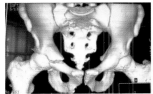 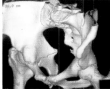 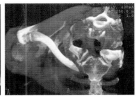

3D imaging is now available. Note the fracture in the right pelvis and the inner end of the clavicle.

Magnetic Resonance Imaging (MRI): Resonance of water molecules in the magnetic field shows soft tissues in vertical and horizontal planes. 3D images are now available. This shows a series of cuts in the sagittal plane of the lumber spine from one side to the other. Note the disc bulge at L4/5.

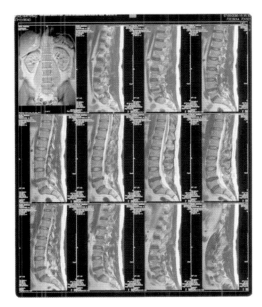

Radio Isotope Scanning: Uptake by bone of isotopes showing hot or cold areas of increased or decreased bone activity. This is normal apart from showing a scoliosis or twist of the spine. The other shows the author's "hot" ankle with inflammation from gouty arthritis.

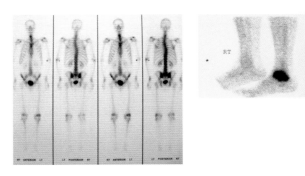

Contrast Medium X-ray: Injection of radio opaque material into a joint shows soft tissue.

Arthroscopy: Looking into a joint.

Arteriography: Injection of radio opaque material into an artery measuring blood flow through an area. Note the pinching of the upper and lower arteries in this arteriogram of a heart. Stents were inserted.

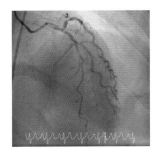

Bone mineral density: Tests where the bones have lost or added calcium.

Electromyography (EMG) or nerve conduction study: tests conductivity of nerves.

Ultrasound: High frequency sound waves show soft tissues.

Having made a diagnosis **treatment** is considered.

The two words that summarise treatment are **kind** and **nous**. To be kind to someone means being gentle and treating them with courtesy and compassion. Nous means using one's common sense and initiative.

Before treatment is commenced the **prognosis** or outcome of the condition must be considered as nature has a strong inbuilt mechanism towards healing and practitioners must assist nature as much as possible.

Results and complications **(side effects)** of treatment must be known. The cure should not be worse than the disease!

General:

The patient must be treated as a whole person and includes not only the management of the acute situation but also convalescence and final recovery.

Local:

Non operative: (or **conservative**) This involves for example the use of drugs e.g analgesics (pain relief), anti-inflammatory (often called NSAIDS-non steroidal anti-inflammatory drugs), massage, manipulation and so on and may be carried out by various disciplines.

Operative: (**surgery**) Pre and post-operative care are as important as the operation itself.

Various suffixes are used to donate operations:

- ostomy/otomy   (cutting into) such as tracheostomy (making a hole in the trachea), osteotomy (cutting into a bone).

- lysis	(freeing of) such as tenolysis (freeing of a tendon), neurolysis (freeing of a nerve)
- ectomy	(removal of) such as gastrectomy (removal of the stomach), appendicectomy (removal of the appendix)
- plasty	(refashioning) such as arthroplasty (making a new joint), mammoplasty (refashioning a breast)
- scopy	(looking into) such as arthroscopy (looking into a joint-arthrus) laparoscopy (looking into the abdomen)
- desis	(fusion) such as arthrodesis (where two bones are fused together and the joint becomes immobile)

Treatment involves a **team** which includes doctors, nurses, physiotherapists, occupational therapists, social workers, osteopaths, chiropractors and paramedical personnel and can take place either at **home** or in **hospital**.

A hospital is like a small city and efficient running requires the help of cooks, porters, engineers, telephonists, secretarial staff, cleaners, gardeners and not least administrators and nowadays security personell.

There is pressure to minimise costs but this must not be allowed to minimise the quality of treatment although costs must be borne in mind.

There is another story from Paré who, towards the end of his career, when he was sent by the King to look after Monsieur le Marquis d'Aurel, a young man who was dying as a result of a compound fracture of the thigh. He wrote in his journal:

"I found him in high fever, his eyes deep sunken, with a moribund and yellowish face, his tongue dry and parched, and the whole body wasted and lean, the voice low, as of a man very near death.

I found his thigh much inflamed, suppurating and ulcerated, discharging a greenish and very offensive sanies. I probed it with a silver probe, wherewith I found a large cavity in the middle of the thigh and others around the knee; also several scales of bone, some loose, others not.

There was a large bedsore; he could rest neither day nor night; and had no appetite to eat, but very thirsty.

Seeing and considering all these great complications and the vital powers thus broken down, truly, I was very sorry I had come to see him because it seemed to me there was very little hope he could escape death.
All the same, to give him courage and good hope, I told him I would soon set him on his legs by the grace of God and the help of his physicians and surgeons.

Having seen him, I went for a walk in the garden, and prayed God to show me this grace, that he should recover, and to bless our hands and our mendicants to cure such a complication of disease. I turned in my mind what measures I must take to this end.

They called me to dinner. I came into the kitchen, and there I saw, taken out of a great pot, half a sheep, a quarter of veal, three great pieces of beef, two fowls, and a very large piece of bacon with abundance of good herbs.

Then I said to myself that the broth of the pot would be full of juices and very nourishing.

After dinner, we began our conversation, all physicians and surgeons together, in the presence of Monsieur le Duc d'Ascot and some other gentleman who were with him. I began to say to the surgeons that I was astonished that they had not made incisions in the patient's thigh, seeing as it was suppurating, and the thick matter in it very foetid and offensive, showing it had long been pent up there; and I had found with the probe caries of the bone and scales of bone already loose.

They answered me, never would he consent to it; and indeed, that it was near two months, since they had been able to get clean sheets on the bed, and that one scare dared to touch the coverlet, so great was his pain.

Then I said, to cure him, we must touch something else than the coverlet of his bed. Each said what he thought of the malady of the patient, and in conclusion they all held it hopeless.

I told them that there was still some hope, because he was young, and God and Nature sometime do what seem to physicians and surgeons impossible.

I proposed three incisions for drainage, fomentations, a clean bed, hot water bottles, a pillow so adjusted as to relieve pressure on the bedsore, dusting powders, an opiate to ensure good sleep at night and a moderate allowance of wine. To help sleep artificial rain must be made by pouring water from a height into a cauldron so that it made the soothing sound of falling rain.

The diet should include raw eggs, plums stewed in wine and sugar, good broth from the pot, fowls and other roast meats easy to digest, good bread that was neither too stale or too new. Medicines prescribed must be properly flavoured, to disguise their taste.

This, my discourse was well approved by the physicians and surgeons. The consultation ended, and we went back to the patient, and I made three openings in his thigh. Two or three hours later, I got a bed made near his old one, with clean white sheets on it; then a strong man put him into it and he was thankful to be taken out of his foul stinking bed.

Soon afterwards, he asked to sleep; which he did for nearly four hours; and everybody in the house began to feel happy ,and especially his brother..........

Then, when I saw him beginning to get well I told him that he was to have viols and violins, and a buffoon to make him laugh; which he did.

In a month, we got him into a chair; and he had himself carried about his garden, and to the door of his Chateau to watch people passing.

The villagers for two or three leagues round, now that they could see him, came on holidays to sing and dance, a regular crowd of light hearted country folk, rejoicing in his convalescence, all glad to see him not without plenty of laughter and plenty of drink. He always gave them a hogshead of beer; and they all drank his health with a will.

In six weeks he began to stand a little on crutches, and to put on flesh and to get a good natural colour. He wanted to go to Beaumont, his brother's place; and was taken thither in a carrying chair; by eight men at a time.

And the peasants, in the villages through which we passed, when they knew it was Monsieur le Marquis fought who should carry him, and insisted that he should drink with them; and it was only beer but they would have given Hippocras, if there had been any; and all were glad to see him, and prayed God for him".

I tell this sorry to emphasise that kindness and common sense will often produce a cure as Paré had himself said " Je l'ai traité, Dieu l'a gueri". (I treated him, God cured him).

These chapters are summarised here and in the back of the book.

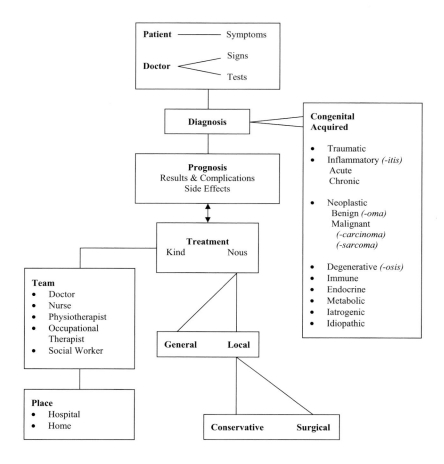

DEVELOPMENTAL DYSPLASIA OF THE HIP (DDH)

This used to be called Congenital Dislocation of the Hip (CDH). The more accepted term is a developmental alteration in the growth of the ball and socket joint. Again there is the use of Latin *dys* meaning faulty and *plasia* meaning growth.

This occurs in about 1/1000 live births and is more commonly seen in females than males in the ratio of 3:1.

Cause

It is thought to be due to laxity of the capsule of the hip possibly due to transfer of hormones across the placental barrier. This causes generalised ligamentous laxity and most babies are able to bring their foot up to their mouth to suck their big toe as easily as they can suck their thumb. They all have flat feet when they first stand up and gradually the arch develops as they grow and the ligaments become stronger.

Most babies have clicking hips at birth but only 1/1000 proceed to a clinical condition. If the hip remains out of socket then changes occur in both the socket and the head of the femur producing a shallow socket or acetabulum and a small head of femur.

Diagnosis in Neonate

Ortolani Test:

The hips are abducted with the knees bent and a click or clunk can be felt and heard as the hip goes in and out of socket. Sometimes there is an alteration in the skin creases in the buttock but this is an inconclusive sign as extra creases are not uncommon.

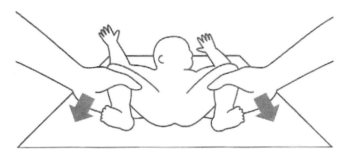

If the condition is suspected an **ultrasound scan** will commonly show whether the hip is in or is out of socket.

Because the bones do not show on x-ray until 3 months of age x-rays are usually not helpful until 3 months of age. They are rarely performed these days.

X-Ray

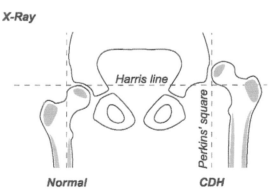

Note the angle the neck makes with the long axis of the femur. This becomes more obtuse as the hip grows in a dislocated hip and is called a **coxa valga**.

Treatment:

Early

Provided the hip is reduced and held within the socket then normal growth will usually resolve the problem. The early treatment is to maintain the hip with the knees out from the side or in **abduction** by the use of double nappies or various forms of harness (Pavlik) or Dennis Brown splints. Sometimes the baby needs to be admitted to hospital for traction with gradual abduction of the hip such that the legs are widely out from the side and when ultrasound or x-rays show the hip is reduced a plaster cast is applied.

Late

If the diagnosis is missed at birth and is not made until the child is walking then surgical treatment is often necessary. Often the child will walk with a waddling gait, or a limp if only one hip is involved. Because the tendons holding the hip in towards the side are tight these are cut by what is called an **adductor tenotomy**. Sometimes the hip is opened and the cartilaginous rim around the hip called the **limbus** is everted to go over the outside of the head of the femur rather than preventing its reduction.

Sometimes it is necessary to alter the shape of the socket through performing an osteotomy or cutting into the pelvis (described by **Salter** of Toronto) and sometimes it is necessary to alter the angle of the neck and shaft of the femur by doing a femoral osteotomy.

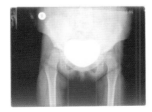
Note the coxa valga on each side. This child was 6 years old with a late diagnosis at two years of age, but then appropriately treated. She was then treated by femoral osteotomy.

Sometimes a dysplastic hip is not diagnosed until the 20s or 30s due to aching in the hip or referred pain to the knee and is picked up on x-ray where there is loss of the neck shaft angle.

The head of the femur is supported by a neck and the angle between the shaft of the femur and the neck is usually 130°. A more open angle alters the forces acting on the hip producing arthritic changes through the surface of the femur and the adjacent acetabulum.

Treatment may be either by femoral osteotomy or more commonly by hip replacement if degenerative change is advanced and the symptoms are severe.

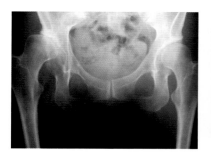 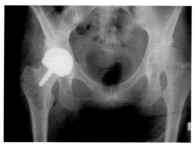

CLUB FEET

This is also called **Congenital Talipes Equio Varus** (CTEV) which means the foot is pointing downwards and inwards. Males are more commonly affected than females in the ratio of 2:1. The calf is often smaller, the heel points inwards and upwards and the foot points downwards with the forefoot swinging towards the midline. If untreated the child can walk but the side of the foot then has to take the pressure of weight bearing as opposed to the sole. It is only seen now in developing countries where there is limited medical access.

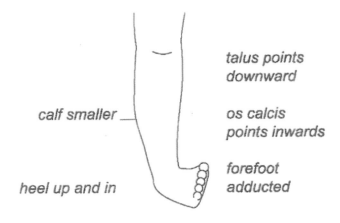

calf smaller

heel up and in

talus points downward

os calcis points inwards

forefoot adducted

Treatment
The aim is to get the foot in a more normal position and the sooner treatment is started the better.

Early

Manipulative   Early treatment is to gently manipulate the foot and do this on a repeated basis and hold the position with strapping or splints or plaster casts. Later Dennis Brown boots can be applied.

Surgical	This is carried out in babies at around 3 months of age which have failed to respond to manipulative treatment. The ligaments on the inner side of the back of the foot are released and the tight heel cord is lengthened, ETA (Elongation Tendo Achilles)
Late	If problems continue or if the child is picked up late bony fusion is necessary where the heel bone and the bone in front of it is fused together (calcaneo-cuboid fusion) carried out between 6 and 9 years of age. A triple arthrodesis is where the three joints at the back of the heel are welded together.

CALCANEO-VALGUS

This is the reverse of club foot and is where the foot points outwards usually due to the way the baby has been lying in utero and no treatment is necessary. Sometimes manipulation is needed but mostly growth will gradually correct the problem.

FLAT FEET (PES PLANUS)

This is due to ligamentous laxity and requires no treatment. The arch can be recreated when the child stands on tiptoes indicating normal function of the joints. Some races have natural flat feet such as the Negroid races and they are the fastest runners in the world. Reassurance of the parents is the best treatment but sometimes insoles are required for the shoes or alteration to the heel of the shoe by lengthening the inner part of the heel. If flat feet are painful the tibialis posterior tendon on the inside of the foot can be advanced and the talo-navicular joint can be fused.

INTOEING

This is common, often associated with the squatting or frog position, and is due to increased internal rotation at the hip. Again growth will usually correct this and reassurance is all that is needed.

CURLY TOES

These are also very common and they are usually in the 3rd and 4th toes where the toes are bent up excessively but no treatment is required. Sometimes if there is pressure, tenotomy of the tendon bending the toes down can be carried out.

KNOCK KNEES & BOW LEGS (GENU VALGUM/GENU VARUM)

This is also common particularly in children who walk early and is due to unequal development of the growth plate at the knee. Mostly they correct as the child grows but sometimes stapling of the growth plate at adolescence is necessary to allow the slower growing side to catch up or, if it is a problem after growth has ceased, an osteotomy is necessary.

SPINA BIFIDA

Because the spine develops from the ectoderm and sinks beneath the skin occasionally this fails to complete and a bulge develops in the lower back which is called a **meningo-myelocoele** or herniations of the spinal cord and

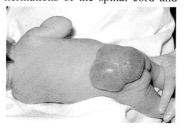

coverings.   This may even be open allowing drainage of the spinal fluid and is often associated with paraplegia. Swelling of the brain due to alteration in the flow of the cerebrospinal fluid is often associated and this is called **hydrocephalus**.

The spinous process of the vertebra develops from either side and if they fail to meet it is called a **bifid spine** and is present normally in the vertebrae of the

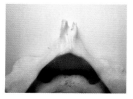

neck (see picture of C5 spine) but abnormally in the lower back and in itself does not cause any problems and is often found by chance on x-ray.

Problems are only noted when it allows herniations of the underlying spinal cord and its coverings. This

is called a **spina bifida overta** whereas the previous is called a **spina bifida occulta**.

Treatment

1.   Close defect
2.   Treat paraplegia in infancy: muscle transfers or callipers
3.   An ileal bladder is necessary
4.   A neurosurgeon performs shunts to allow free drainage of the cerebrospinal fluid

CEREBRAL PALSY

This occurs in about 1/1000 births and is due to brain damage from various causes such as lack of oxygen, trauma, jaundice or infection. Brain function is usually not affected and the child is of normal or above average intelligence.

Spastic   This is where the muscles contract uncontrollably and may produce a scissor gait or tense muscles.

Athetoid   Is where there is variation in the way the muscles contract allowing writhing movements

Treatment

Treatment is by splints, muscle transfers or tenotomies and treatment in a normal school if the child is not grossly affected, otherwise in a special school where more nursing care is required.

MUSCLE DYSTROPHIES

This where the muscle fails to function properly, and because of paralysis of the respiratory muscles death can occur from associated infection of the lung.

ACHONDROPLASIA

This is a condition where the normal growth of the bones is inhibited and a person developes a short stature (a dwarf) with a normal sized head but short arms and legs and a short body.

OSTEOGENESIS IMPERFECTA

This is a condition where the bones are more fragile and is associated with collagen and calcium deficiency in bones producing brittle bones. The collagen deficiency allows the darkness of the retina to shine through such that the white in the eye appears blue.

Treatment

Treat fractures as they occur and this may involve preventative treatment such as rodding of the femora and tibiae.

OSTEOCHONDRITIS

1. Crushing

The blood supply to a part is cut off (tissue **necrosis**). The dead bone erodes and is gradually replaced (**creeping substitution**).

Perthes Disease (hip)

	(Ages 5-10, boys > girls)
Symptoms	Pain, often in the knee. Limp
Signs	"Irritable" hip. Decreased abduction of the hip
Tests	Blood tests and x-rays are often all normal initially. X-ray change develops later with porosis and sclerosis, flattening of the head (mushroom effect) and in older patients the "sagging rope" sign.

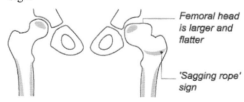

The effects depend on the amount of head of the femur involved and the age of onset. The earlier the onset and the smaller the amount of head involved the better the prognosis.

43

Treatment

1. Bed rest for the irritable hip for two to three weeks
2. Surgery – Innominate osteotomy to provide cover for the femoral head

Scheuermann's disease (spine)

(Ages 12-17, boys > girls)

Symptoms   Backache usually in the thoracic spine

Signs   Increased kyphosis (adolescent kyphosis)

Tests   X-rays may show wedging of the vertebral bodies.   Schmorl's nodes (disc intrusion into the bodies)

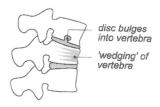

disc bulges
into vertebra

'wedging' of
vertebra

Treatment

1. Exercises
2. Brace

2. Splitting *Dissecans*: Part of the articular surface separates. Common in the knee (13-14, boys > girls)

Less common elbow, ankle

Symptoms   Pain in the joint, clicking or locking

Signs   Often normal examination

Tests   X-rays show separate fragment or loose body

Treatment

Arthroscopy and fix if possible with wires or screws, or excise

3. Pulling   Where a tendon pulls on an apophysis (part of the growth plate) producing inflammation (apophysitis)

Osgood-Schlatter's (knee) This is the author's adult knee showing the separated fragment of the apophysis.

(13-15, boys > girls)

Sever's (heel) (9-13, girls > boys)

Symptoms   Pain

Signs   Local tenderness

Prominent tibial tubercle

Tests   X-rays sometimes show a separate ossicle in the tibial apophysis, fragmentation of the calcaneal apophysis.

Treatment

Most settle when growth ceases.

1. *Restrict activity:* Football in boys, ballet in girls
2. *Surgery:*   Excise bony fragment

SLIPPED EPIPHYSIS (SUFE - slipped upper femoral epiphysis)

Boys more than girls – 10-15, fat boys or tall and thin, 40% bilateral; always x-ray both hips.

      a)   Acute

      b)   General

Symptoms   Pain in hip or knee

                Limp

Signs   The hip goes into external rotation on flexion

Tests   X-ray shows disordered Trethowan's line, Shenton's arc, parrot's beak

                (chronic)

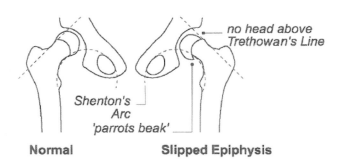

Normal   **Slipped Epiphysis**

Treatment   Reduce if possible. Internally fix. Beware chondrolysis and early onset osteoarthritis

SCOLIOSIS

Deviation of the spine from the normal vertical alignment

Cause: **Secondary** to

a) neuromuscular disorders e.g. polio

b) infection e.g. TB

c) degeneration

Idiopathic

Commonest; female > males; teenagers

Symptoms   Prominence on the back noted, often on school examination

Signs   Lateral deviation and rotation of spine with rib hump on flexion (hunchback)

Tests   *X-ray:* Standing views. Angle noted in primary curve (Cobb).

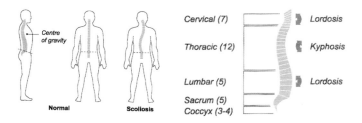

Treatment:Conservative

a) Exercises

b) Splintage

- Milwaukee brace

- Risser jacket

Surgical   Curve > 40 degrees Spinal fusion with some form of internal fixation

ACUTE OSTEOMYELITIS

This is common in young children and the infection comes via the blood stream
to the growing end of the bone (metaphysis). It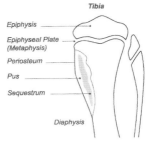
often does not spread into the epiphysis due to
the adherence of the periosteum and
cartilaginous plate of the metaphysis. It may
spread into the shaft or diaphysis of the bone.
Acute inflammation and pus formation follows.
The pus is forced out beneath the periosteum
and may spread along the shaft and around it. It may burst into the bone or out
through the soft tissues. The commonest organism is Staphylococcus aureus.

Because periosteum makes new bone when it is lifted off a whole new shaft of
the bone may form as in the following x-rays of the author's left leg, as a baby
prior to the invention of antibiotics.

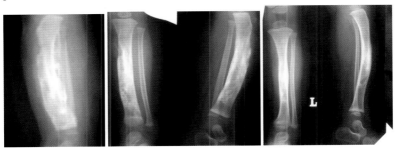

Note the new shaft developing, the loss of the old, with a successful outcome.

Symptoms: The child is ill and in acute pain

Signs: There is fever due to septicaemia or the spread of organisms through the blood stream. Movement is possible at the joint but the child resists movement. If there is an infection in the joint movement is not possible. This is called a septic arthritis.

Tests: *Culture* of the blood is taken and a full blood screen shows a raised white count and a raised sedimentation rate.

X-rays: No changes are seen initially but later new bone is noted beneath the elevated periosteum.

Treatment:

Conservative:

The child is treated with bed rest and antibiotics with broad spectrum antibiotics given initially until the offending organism is found. The affected limb is splinted.

Surgical:

Surgical treatment involves early drainage and this may involve drilling the bone to release the pus which is often under pressure.

Complications and results:

Most cases now recover fully but occasionally some go on to chronic osteomyelitis where there is recurrent infection and this may occur even some years later. Sometimes the organisms set up a happy hunting ground in other places and form what is called metastatic abscesses. Chronic inflammation of the lining of the bone or periostitis forms and occasionally there is chronic inflammation in the muscles known as myositis.

CHRONIC OSTEOMYELITIS

This is a chronic inflammation usually due to an underlying sequestrum. This may be an area of bone that has lost its blood supply by acute infection or following a fracture or post surgery. Sometimes the presence of a foreign body such as a screw or a joint replacement may be present, producing an irritation and further reaction and infection. Pus escapes through a sinus. The organism is often resistant to antibiotics and the commonest organism is MRSA (Methicillin Resistant Staphylococcus Aureus). Sometimes no organism is grown especially when there has been extensive antibiotic treatment.

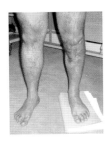 Scars tethered to bone are indications of previous osteomyelitis or healed infection. This was a complicated case with an open fracture requiring skin grafting and there was resultant shortening of the leg. He is standing on his thick file of notes which evens up the leg length discrepancy.

Symptoms: There is pain and a discharge

Signs: The skin is thickened, scaly and red and there is a sinus present with the discharge of pus.

Tests: *X-ray:* The bone is thickened with osteosclerosis and porosis present. A lucent line is seen around an implant if present.

Culture: Shows organisms and sensitivity

Treatment:

Conservative:

The treatment is by rest and antibiotics

Surgical:

Drainage is often necessary together with irrigation and removal of the offending area of dead bone or the prosthesis. Sometimes an immediate replacement can be carried out provided there is strong antibiotic cover. If the fracture has not united it may be necessary to change to an external fixation device. The bone can be saucerised and occasionally in chronic cases with complications, amputation is considered.

ACUTE SEPTIC ARTHRITIS

This is due to infection within the joint and the child has similar signs and symptoms to acute osteomyelitis except there is no movement possible in the joint.

Treatment:

The treatment is systemic antibiotics and aspiration and injection of antibiotics into the joint itself. Immediate surgical treatment is essential to prevent damage to the lining articular cartilage.

Complications:

If immediate treatment is not successful cartilage necrosis may occur and arthritis develops in the joint. This is more likely if the infection becomes chronic.

POLIOMYELITIS

Unfortunately this is still common in underdeveloped countries. It is due to a virus affecting the anterior horn cells in the spinal column producing paralysis of various muscles. It has been prevented by oral or intradermal vaccination since the 1950s and is rarely found in developed countries now. The consequences are due to the weakness of muscles.

Muscle strength is assessed by the following table:

0	Total paralysis
1	Flicker
2	Contraction but no strong enough to overcome gravity
3	Strong enough to overcome gravity
4	Strong but not normal
5	Normal

Child affected:

The growth is retarded, the limb is shortened and thin and there is atrophic skin and thin bones.

Treatment:
Conservative:

Splintage: Callipers, built up shoe

Surgical:

a)   Leg lengthening

b)   Tendon transfers

c)   Joint fusion if there is a dropped foot.

TUBERCULOSIS

This again is uncommon in developed countries but common in developing countries. Unfortunately the organism of the tubercle bacillus has become resistant to antibiotics and is now recurrent particularly in the lower socio-economic group who fail to finish their course of treatment or get lost to follow up. The bacillus infects the lung and the lymph nodes and is spread to the bones and joints by the blood stream. It can be prevented by BCG vaccination. It used to be common in infected dairy herds producing infected milk.

General effects: Night sweats and weight loss

Local effects: The joint is usually swollen and there is associated muscle wasting and stiffness. There is increased kyphosis in the spine and it used to be called Pott's disease or spinal tuberculosis (see page 81).

Treatment:

Conservative:

The treatment of tuberculosis is by drugs: Rifampicin

Isoniazid

Ethambutol

Streptomycin

Pyrazinamide

Surgical:

The surgical treatment is to drain the abscess or irrigate the joint and remove the synovial membrane

Complications:

Stiffness in the joint due to scarring, sinus formation and late recurrence

FRACURES AND DISLOCATIONS

The cause is a force either applied directly or indirectly. The degree of damage depends on the amount of force applied and the resilience of the tissues.

Bone is **hard** tissue and a **fracture** is a break in a bone.

There is also damage to **soft** tissues such as bruising, haematoma or laceration and grazing of the skin.

A **sprain** is a stretching of the ligaments and a **subluxation** is a joint partially out of socket where the capsule is torn and a **dislocation** is where the joint is fully out of socket.

Pathological fractures may occur with minimal force indicating underlying disease such as osteoporosis or metastatic deposits from carcinoma or sarcoma. **Stress (fatigue) fractures** occur following repetitive minor force and are commonly called shin splints in the leg, or, march fractures in the foot.

Types:

1. **Closed** or **open** with perforation of the overlying soft tissues from within or without.

2. **Simple** or **complicated** involving vessels and nerves. There is always soft tissue damage associated and this affects the outcome.

3. They are classified according to the appearance of the bone ends at the fracture site and fracture description relates to the distal fragment (angulation or rotation). Various classifications are used.

Fractures

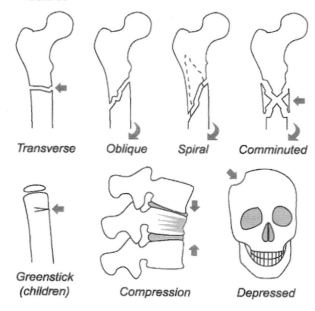

Transverse   Oblique   Spiral   Comminuted

Greenstick
(children)   Compression   Depressed

Symptoms: Pain and loss of function

Signs: Are the same as for inflammation with deformity, swelling, bruising and tenderness and often crepitus at the fracture site.

Tests: Involves x-rays, MRI, CT scans and ultrasound

Treatment:

AIM: Complete and early restoration of function. Before treatment can be considered it is important to know:

     Site   Where the fracture is

     Type   The type of fracture

     Displacement   Seen on x-ray on 2 views AP and lateral e.g. impacted, angulated, rotated. Remember the description relates to the distal fragment.

General:

1. First aid and transport to the hospital or surgery
2. Pain relief
3. Blood replacement if necessary

Local:

REDUCE   *Restore to correct alignment by:*

     a) Closed manipulation which is the art of orthopaedics or good bone setting which orthopaedic surgeons used to be called.

     b) Open reduction (if closed impossible or inaccurate). Not all fractures require reduction and a poor position in children can be accepted as growth will correct the deformity, but not rotational deformity as shown in the following pictures.

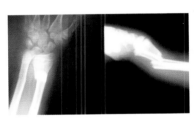 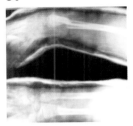

Unfortunately young surgeons find it difficult to resist operating on such a fracture. There are really only two fractures in children that demand open reduction and these are fractures of the lateral epicondyle in the elbow and fractures of the surgical neck of the femur.

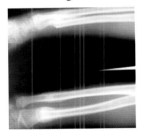 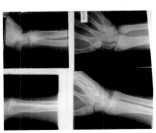

Note union has occurred at six weeks and by one year it is difficult to see where the bone has been broken.

HOLD   *This is only necessary if the fracture is unstable or potentially unstable*

a)   By   plaster   (as   shown   above),   splintage   or   traction.

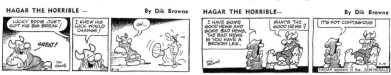

b) By internal fixation with screws, wires, pins and nails, and again one has to be aware of the pitfalls of surgery. **ORIF (open reduction internal fixation).**

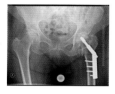

c) A combination such as the use of an external fixator first pioneered by Ilazarov and this is particularly useful in open fractures.

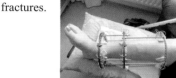

USE   **The most important aspect of treatment** is to maintain and restore function.   It involves exercising muscles and joints not immobilised with the aid of **physiotherapy.** Note the knee bending even with the fixator in place

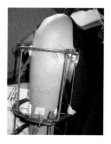

HEALING OF FRACTURES/TISSUES

Healing is progressive and commences immediately. A good blood supply is essential for proper healing. It is divided into stages but is a continuous process.

Stage 1

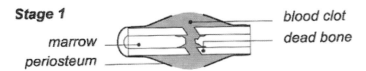

Haematoma: as bone bleeds a clot (haematoma) forms between the broken ends. Bruising and swelling may be seen.

Stage 2

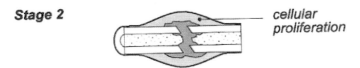

Cellular proliferation: Fibroblasts, chondroblasts, osteoblasts and macrophages invade the haematoma over the succeeding 10 days. An increased blood supply is established.

Stage 3

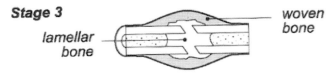

Callus: Woven bone is formed and calcification starts to occur over the next 4-6 weeks allowing the fracture to become firm.

Stage 4

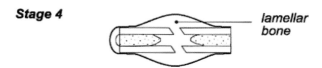

lamellar
bone

Consolidation: Lamella bone is formed and bone is laid down in lines of stress. This takes several months. Clinical union occurs during this phase.

Stage 5

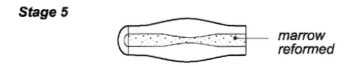

marrow
reformed

Remodelling: The bone is restored as nearly as possible to the original and this process can take up to two years.

Direct healing is seen in rigid internal fixation with no obvious callus. Indirect healing where there is some movement at the fracture ends shows callus.

Clinical union is defined when the bone is stable on examination. **Radiological union** is defined when the fracture is consolidated on x-ray. MRI scans unfortunately are often misinterpreted as showing non union of a fracture when there is both clinical and radiological union due to the amount of water present at the fracture site. Healing of fractures could be likened to the setting of concrete where the chemical processes allow hardening over a few hours and then curing over several months or years. It is said that the Hoover Dam, one of the largest concrete structures in the world built in the 1930s, is still curing.

Time: Children get half price so they get half the time

	Spiral fracture	Transverse
Upper limb	6 weeks	12 weeks
Lower limb	12 weeks	24 weeks

Factors affecting healing:

There are various factors that can affect healing including the age of the patient and their general health. The local effects are:

1. Degree of local trauma
2. Degree of bone loss
3. Type of bone (compact, cancellous)
4. Degree of stability
5. Infection
6. Involvement of joint (synovial fluid)
7. Presence of local malignancy
8. Radiation necrosis

Complications: There are general complications and local complications.

General:

1. **Shock** due to loss of blood and fluids, or hypovolaemia, and the treatment is with fluid and blood replacement

2. **Crush syndrome** where muscles are destroyed and release a toxin resulting in renal failure and occurs commonly with fallen masonry and earthquakes. The treatment is to resect the muscles or even amputation, and kidney dialysis.

3. **Fat embolism**. This occurs with long bone fractures and is due to the release of fatty acids into the blood stream setting up an inflammation of the lung or pneumonitis. It occurs in the first few days following injury. Hypoxia results in increased respiratory rate, increased heart rate and cerebral confusion. Sometimes there is an elevated temperature and petechial haemorrhages or tiny little spots of blood can be seen in the skin or in the eyes. Test: blood gases show low arterial oxygen, and the **treatment** is with oxygen and steroids.

4. **Deep vein thrombosis (DVT) and pulmonary embolism (PE).** This occurs when there is sluggish circulation through the veins allowing clots to form in the deep veins. Breaking off of these clots travelling to the lungs causes pulmonary embolism, and can be fatal. **Treatment** is best by prophylaxis with exercises, elevation of the limbs and low molecular weight heparin. Once the condition has been diagnosed it is necessary to anticoagulate the patient with heparin and Warfarin.

Local complications:

1. **Bone**

    a) *Delayed union:* This is due to a poor blood supply with a large gap and excessive movement and infection. It is common in tubular bones where there is thick cortex and little cancellous bone such as the clavicle and tibia.

    b) *Non-union:* Occurs where the callus is replaced by scar tissue-**(pseudarthrosis)**.

    Treatment of delayed and non union is by electrical stimulation, high frequency sound waves or lithotrypsy and bone grafting, bringing in bone cells from, for example, the pelvic crest. Sometimes all that is necessary is to freshen the bone ends and internally fix a fracture. If there are screws used in rods for e.g. the tibia the top or bottom screws can be removed to allow the bone to slide along the rod (**dynamisation**).

    c) *Mal-union:* This occurs when the fracture is allowed to join in a faulty position either by inadequate reduction or fixation. It can sometimes be accepted but otherwise is treated by osteotomy. Shortening may occur.

    d) *Avascular necrosis:* This occurs when the blood supply is interrupted particularly in the neck of the femur or the waist of the scaphoid.

    e) *Osteoporosis:* This is due to disuse and patients must be encouraged to weight bear if possible and undertake an exercise programme.

Sometimes a condition called **Complex Regional Pain Syndrome** may occur where there is alteration in the blood supply and nerve supply producing pain and skin sensation changes.

f) *Prominent metal ware:* This is seen when a plate and screws, for example, is used to fix a clavicle fracture and the screw heads become prominent requiring removal once the fracture has joined.

2.   Joint

Stiffness is the commonest complication usually due to prolonged immobilisation and lack of exercise in the joints not immobilised. Once it develops it is treated by physiotherapy and sometimes manipulation under anaesthetic. It is best prevented by encouraging exercise from the beginning. The patient must be reassured that they will do no harm and to move even if it hurts. Osteoarthritis occurs when the joint surface has been damaged.

3.   Soft tissue damage

Soft tissues are always involved in fractures and sometimes specific damage occurs to, for example, nerves in some situations such as a humeral fracture involving the radial nerve or vessels such as the popliteal artery behind the knee, or muscles. These become wasted due to disuse. There is a condition called the **Compartment Syndrome** where swelling in the muscles affects the blood supply producing intense pain. It is diagnosed by measuring the compartmental pressure and the treatment is by emergency fasciotomy. The late result is scarring in the muscle producing contracture such as **Volkmann's contracture** or clawing of the hand or foot.

4.   Infection

This is common following open fractures or surgery and the treatment is as for osteomyelitis with antibiotics and wound debridement.

THE MANAGEMENT OF MAJOR ACCIDENTS

1.   The management at scene and transport to hospital: This is usually left to the paramedics who arrive but prior to their arrival it is important to **establish an airway** to maintain respiration and to **arrest bleeding**. The spinal cord should be protected by keeping the patient still until a hard collar can be applied and a spinal board fitted.

2.   Treatment in Accident and Emergency: The ATLS (Advanced Trauma and Life Support) system is followed. (EMST - early management of severe trauma - in Australasia)

    Primary survey:

    A Airway (cervical spine control)

    B Breathing and ventilation

    C Circulation. Control haemorrhage. Blood pressure. Pulse. An i.v.(intra-venous) cannula is inserted and fluids commenced to prevent shock

    D Disability (neurological status)

        A   Alert

        V   Responds to vocal stimuli

        P   Responds to painful stimuli

        U   Unconscious

    E Exposure (undress patient, keep warm)

    R Resuscitate

    Secondary survey:

    History

    Examination: including Glasgow Coma Scale (GCS). Normal (15)

- Eye opening (4)
- Verbal response (5)
- Motor response (6)

    Treatment: Repair damage – **Priorities**: Ruptured spleen takes precedence over fractured femur

FRACTURES AND DISLOCATIONS IN THE UPPER LIMB

Function is important: Do not immobilise too long

Fractured clavicle: Very common. Union good. Figure 8 for 3 weeks
or sling only. Warn mother of lump of callus in child

Dislocation Acromio-clavicular (AC) joint:

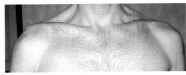 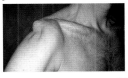 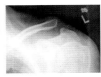

Internal fixation plate needs removal 3-6 months later.
The x-rays are from a different patient.

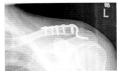

Fractured scapula: Sling for a few days

Fractured neck of humerus: Common.   Elderly   patients.   Impacted
fracture. Sling for 2 weeks under clothes then exercise

Dislocated shoulder: Common anterior
Reduce: Kocher manoeuvre (traction, externally rotate,
                                adduct, internally rotate).   Hippocratic (foot in
                                axilla, pull and adduct)
Hold: Sling/body bandage 3-6 weeks
Use: Exercises

Recurrent dislocation: Common, requires surgery, fix detached labrum
Fracture shaft humerus: Collar and cuff sling and gravity.   POP splints
                                ORIF often needed.

Supracondylar: Common in children. Always admit; watch for arterial damage. Gross swelling. If necessary traction in extension. Mal-union produces gunstock deformity.

Fractured neck & head of radius: Excise if comminuted. Exercise

Fractured olecranon: Gap fracture, reduce – hold by internal fixation

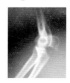 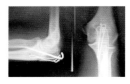

Dislocated elbow: Reduce. Stable. Sling for few days

Fractured radius & ulna (both bones): Difficult to hold, often best to operate

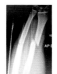 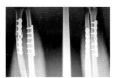

Fractured radius & dislocated ulna: At wrist – Galliazzi

Fractured ulna & dislocated radius: At elbow – Monteggia

Always make sure both elbow and wrist joints are included in the x-ray if there is a single bone fracture. Open reduction nearly always necessary

Colles fracture: This was first described by Abraham Colles in 1814 (1773-1843) which he did without the benefit of x-rays. Very common. Fall on outstretched hand.

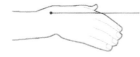
*Dinner Fork Deformity
(Radial deviation, dorsal
displacement, backward
angulation, comminution)*

Reduce: Traction on thumb and index finger, pronate, ventrally displace

Hold: POP cast 4-6 weeks. Re x-ray in 1 week as often redisplaces
  N.B *Advise exercises. Shoulder, elbow and fingers*

Smith's fracture/Barton's fracture: Reversed Colles. May require open reduction and fixation with buttress plate

Fractured scaphoid: Common. Blood supply may be affected. If suspected (tender anatomical snuffbox) POP cast, re x-ray 1 week, 10 days. Cast 6-8 weeks, may require screw fixation

Dislocation of wrist (lunate): Often missed. CT scan if unsure. Open reduction often necessary

Fractured metacarpals: Usually no fixation. Exercise fingers

Fractured base 1st metacarpal: (Bennett's fracture). Abduct thumb, may require open reduction

Skier's, biker's thumb: This used to be called gamekeeper's thumb and is a rupture of the ligament on the inner side of the metacarpophalangeal joint due to forced abduction of the thumb.

Fractured neck 5th metacarpal: Boxer's fracture. Difficult to hold, not reduced, exercise fingers

Fractured phalanges: Strap to adjacent finger

PIP (proximal inter-phalangeal) dislocation: Commonly seen in cricketers where the ball strikes the outstretched finger. Reduce. Exercise.

Mallet finger: Rupture extensor tendon or base of distal phalanx. Splint 6 weeks. Occasionally repair tendon

FRACTURES AND SPRAINS OF THE SPINE

Spinal injuries may be:

    1.   Stable

    2.   Unstable – beware cord damage

Mechanism of injury: Falls. Sport (rugby). Lifting. Motor Vehicle Accident (MVA). Falling masonry (bombs, earthquakes).

Types:

1.	*Extension*	Chip fracture off anterior longitudinal ligament (Avulsion fractures)
2.	*Flexion*	Crush or wedge compression fracture
3.	*Compression*	Straight spine, burst fracture
4.	*Rotation*	Plus combination of flexion

- unstable – may produce dislocation of facet joints
- unstable – cord at risk

STABLE FRACTURES AND SPRAINS

CERVICAL SPINE

1. **Soft tissue injury or muscular ligamentous sprain**

This is common following rear impact motor vehicle accidents and **whiplash** is a term commonly used. It is more the mechanism of injury which is a backward and forward jolt of the head on the neck. The backward movement of the head is now prevented by the headrest and the forward movement by the chin hitting the chest. Since sash belts have been introduced whiplash injuries have become more common. In a rear shunt the vehicle that is struck is called the **target** vehicle and the striking vehicle a **bullet** vehicle. Because the bullet vehicle is at fault legally it is interesting to note that the victims of the target vehicle are the ones that develop symptoms whereas the mechanism of injury is the same. It is similarly noted that when cars are stationary and somebody reverses into a target vehicle again it is the **victim** that complains of symptoms. Litigation has been shown to prolong symptoms and often they do not resolve after completion of the case. The muscles most commonly involved are the muscles in the back of the neck but sometimes also in drivers the muscles of the rotator cuff can be involved producing pain on lifting the arm from the side. Airbags were invented to prevent forward jolting of the body as Americans do not like wearing seatbelts. Symptoms develop even in low velocity accidents.

2. **Wedge, crush or compression fractures**

Symptoms: Pain; neck, back of shoulder (trapezius)

Down arm (brachialgia)

Headache

Stiffness

Signs: Restricted movements. Wry neck

Tests: *X-ray* - often normal or may show loss of lordosis in sprains. Wedge shaped vertebra in fractures.

MRI – may show disc lesion but often present in normal population as degeneration commences in the twenties and increases linearly with age. It is not necessarily symptomatic.

CT - in presence of fracture to determine if cord threatened

EMG – assess peripheral nerves in arm

Treatment:

General
a) Analgesics or painkillers
b) Anti-inflammatory drugs particularly slow release drugs
c) Relaxants such as diazepam in the first two weeks or in chronic symptoms amitriptyline, a mild tranquillizer that is taken at night

Local
a) A collar is often useful for the first 1 - 2 weeks although exercise is more commonly recommended now. A soft pillow is helpful
b) Physiotherapy – traction, ultrasound, short wave diathermy, TENS machine (Transcutaneous Electrical Nerve Stimulation), hydrotherapy, massage
c) **Exercises** such as swimming, cycling, rowing, exercise at a gym, Pilates, yoga, walking, dancing and posture all help
d) Manipulation with or without anaesthetic
e) Chiropractic
f) Osteopathy
g) Acupuncture
h) Alternative therapy e.g. Aromatherapy, Naturopathy, Bowen, Reflexology, Hypnotherapy
i) Trigger point injections, facet joint injections often under the supervision of a pain clinic

The majority of patients with neck sprains recover within six months but recovery can take as long as 3 years and some are left with permanent symptoms. Studies have shown no acceleration of spondylosis or degenerative change, which renders the spine more susceptible to a spraining injury.

THORACIC/LUMBAR SPINE

1.   **Low back sprain**

Soft tissue injury, muscular ligamentous sprain, facet joint sprain.   Usually after heavy lifting.

(Disc injury see Spinal disorders – page 92)

2.   **Compression fracture**

Wedge, crush. Usually after fall, spontaneous in elderly osteoporotic women

Symptoms:	Pain
	Stiffness
Signs:	Reduced movement, especially flexion
	Kyphus, Dowager hump
Tests:	*X-ray* – Loss of lordosis in sprains

Wedging of anterior vertebra in fractures, as shown in the author's old Lumbar 1 vertebral fracture with associated degeneration.

Generalised osteoporosis.

Osteolysis (metastatic deposit).

Blood – Acid phosphatase if prostatic secondary suspected (raised).   Alkaline phosphatase if lung, breast secondary suspected (raised)

Treatment

General: a)   Bed rest

             b)   Fracture board

             c)   Drugs; analgesics, anti-inflammatories, relaxants

Local: a)   Corset, brace, plaster jacket

            b)   Physiotherapy

            c)   Exercises, swimming

Complications:

            a)   Urinary retention

            b)   Constipation

            c)   Stiffness, may need manipulation

SPONDYLOLYSIS

Defect in pas interarticularis. Often asymptomatic.

Tests: X-ray -   oblique   -   **'Scotty Dog'** *(oblique view)*

          Scotty dog   collar

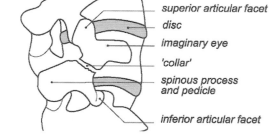

- superior articular facet
- disc
- imaginary eye
- 'collar'
- spinous process and pedicle
- inferior articular facet

SPONDYLOLISTHESIS

Seen in 5% of the population.

Grade 1-4 forward displacement of vertebra. May be asymptomatic. If symptomatic: Back pain +/- sciatica

Treat: Brace, Exercises and physiotherapy, Spinal fusion if severe and symptomatic.

UNSTABLE FRACTURES AND FRACTURE DISLOCATIONS

CERVICAL, THORACIC, LUMBAR SPINES

Immediate management important to end result

1. Transport to Spinal Injuries Unit without delay
2. Take care to avoid further injury.   Stabilise spine until properly assessed: Hard collar. Spinal board
3. Maintain airway and ventilation

Cord damage

In 40% of cervical fractures, 5% thoracic/lumbar.

Lateral cervical spine x-ray (all 7 and T1) mandatory in all patients sustaining an injury above the clavicle.

Signs:	1.	Spinal shock:	Loss of sensation
			Loss of reflexes
	2.	Return of muscle function and spasms, rigidity (days to weeks later)	

Quadriplegia:	Paralysis all four limbs
	(Christopher Reeve, Superman)
Paraplegia:	Paralysis lower limbs
Hemiplegia:	Paralysis of one side of the body (due to cerebrovascular accident/stroke)

Treatment:

1. *Reduce*	Open reduction if necessary
2. *Hold*	Skull traction (Crutchfield tongs
	Spinal fusion
3. *Good nursing*	Essential. Applies to any patient especially elderly

a) **Skin:**   *Anaesthetic skin develops pressure sores within hours*

- No creases in sheets; no crumbs in bed
- 2 hourly turning
- Wash and dry skin carefully
- Use powder and oil
- Adjust pillows
- Spinal beds – ripple mattresses
- Turning beds, moving patient helped if spine fused

b) **Bladder:**   *Avoid infection (ultimately leads to renal failure and death)*

- Catherisation – strict asepsis
- Change weekly
- Antiseptics, antibiotics
- Train bladder by filling and emptying

c) **Bowel:**   *Avoid constipation*

- Train by aperients, enemas
- Abdominal exercises

d) **Muscles and joints:**   *Avoid contractures*

- Physiotherapy
- Passive stretching

e) **Morale:**   *Avoid depression*

- Role model (Christopher Reeve)
- Occupational therapy
- Special workshops
- Sports (Paralympics)

FRACTURES OF THE PELVIS

1. *PELVIC RING FRACTURES*

Displacement slight. Complications rare

Treatment: Rest, analgesics, mobilise when pain allows

2. *PELVIC RING DISRUPTIONS*

Displacement severe, large blood loss

Complications common:

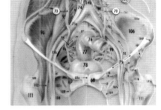

a) Genito-urinary tears

b) Iliac vessel tears

Treatment:

Reduce: Traction, Open reduction and fixation

Repair: Soft tissue injury

Combined surgical approach depends on tissue damage

3. *AVULSION FRACTURES*

Treatment: Mobilise when comfortable

4. *SACROCOCCYGEAL INJURIES*

Coccydynia

Treatment: Avoid sitting in acute phase

Ring cushion

Injection of local anaesthetic and steroid

Excise coccyx (coccygectomy). However results of surgery are variable

FRACTURES AND DISLOCATIONS IN LOWER LIMB

1. *FRACTURES IN FEMORAL NECK:*

a) Subcapital (intracapsular)

60-70 age group

b) Intertrochanteric (extracapsular)

70-80 age group. More common
in females as they outlive men

c) Subtrochanteric

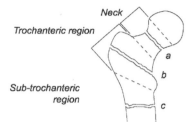

Signs: Leg short, externally rotated

Important queries as they affect length of stay

a) Could patient walk before

b) Home circumstances. Activities of Daily Living (ADL)

c) Mental state

In general patient moves down i.e. If independent goes to live with relative; if there already goes to a nursing home.

Treatment: Principles apply: ***Reduce:*** All require operation, and as patient is often frail, operate as soon as possible.

Hold: a) Subcapital, Garden type 1-4 (depends on displacement).

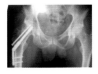

1-2 (mild) Internal fixation with compression screws

3,4 (severe) Replace femoral head
(Moore's, Thompson's prosthesis)

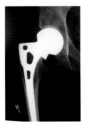

b)   Intertrochanteric, Dynamic Hip Screw (DHS)

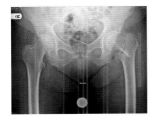 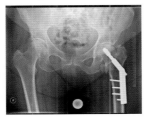

c)   Subtrochanteric, Intramedullary rod e.g. Russell Taylor nail

This was a difficult fracture as the hip was previously fused, and the initial plate and screws failed requiring the subsequent revision to an intra-medullary nail.

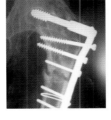 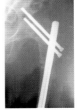

Use: Commence walking as soon as possible

Complications:

1.   Delayed union, non-union

2.   Avascular necrosis (30% Garden 3,4 therefore primary replacement)

3.   DVT and pulmonary embolism

4.   50% of patients die within 2 years because they are old, and have concomitant disease.

2. **DISLOCATION OF HIP**

    a)   **Posterior** common, blow on knee. Hip flexed, leg adducted, internally rotated but beware concomitant fracture shaft when leg lies in external rotation

    b)   **Anterior**. Leg abducted externally rotated

    c)   **Medial**. Fracture pelvis (floor of acetabulum)

Treatment:

Reduce: Under general anaesthetic by manipulation, or open reduction and internal fixation.

Hold: By traction

Use: Exercise

3.   *FEMORAL SHAFT FRACTURE:*

1-2 litre blood loss, high, low

    a)   Transverse

    b)   Oblique

    c)   Comminuted

Treatment:

Conservative: **Traction**: Skin, Skeletal - pin through proximal tibia, Ropes, pulleys and weights. Various: Perkins, Hamilton Russell, Thomas splint

Operative:

    Intramedullary nailing under image intensifier control, with interlocking screws

4. **_FRACTURES INTO KNEE JOINT_**

Aspirate haemarthrosis. Accurate reduction. Internal fixation. Beware popliteal artery damage; vascular surgeon on hand or transfer to centre with vascular unit.

5. **_PATELLAR FRACTURES_**

a) _Intact extensor mechanism (no gap)_

Aspirate haemarthrosis, minimal support, active exercises

b) _Displaced._ Open reduction and tension band wiring. Patellectomy if comminuted (repair extensor quadriceps mechanism)

6. **_LIGAMENT TEARS_**

Medial, lateral, cruiciates – increased "play", positive drawer sign. MRI helpful

Treatment
Conservative: Aspirate haemarthrosis, Cast or splint, Physiotherapy

Surgical: a) Open repair medial or lateral

b) Late reconstruction Anterior Cruciate Ligament (ACL)

7. **_RECURRENT DISLOCATION PATELLA_**

Common in teenage girls. Lateral dislocation (altered anatomical slope) lax ligaments

Treatment

Conservative: Strengthen quadriceps

Surgical: Realign patellar tendon

8.   *TIBIAL FRACTURES*

Proximal, middle, lower third

    a)   Transverse

    b)   Spiral or oblique

    c)   Comminuted

    d)   Fatigue (shin splints)

High ratio cortical bone therefore delayed, non-union likely.   Beware compartment syndrome – Fasciotomy all four

Treatment

Conservative:

Reduce: Manipulation under GA

Hold: Plaster or fibre cast

Use: Crutches: non or partial weight bearing (NWB, PWB)

Surgical: Elevation on Braun frame with calcaneal pin traction to reduce swelling for 2 weeks if comminuted and very swollen. Intramedullary nailing with proximal and distal locking screws. Reamed nailing promotes osteoblastic activity

9.   *ANKLE*

    a)   *Sprains.* Lateral ligament common. If total tear suspected - stress inversion x-ray. May require open repair

Treatment: Ice

    Strapping

    Physiotherapy

b)   *Fractures.* Inversion and eversion with rotation. Medical and/or lateral and/or posterior malleoli. Various classifications (used to be called Pott's fractures after Percival Pott. He lived from 1714 to 1788 and wrote numerous articles whilst laid up following a fracture of his ankle when he was thrown from his horse in 1758. His son-in-law writes: *Conscious of the dangers attendant on fractures of this nature and thoroughly aware how much they may be increased by rough treatment or improper position he would not suffer himself to be moved until he had made the necessary disposition. He sent to Westminster for two chairmen to bring their poles; the patient lay on the cold pavement, it being the middle of January until they arrived. In this situation he purchased a door to which he made them nail their poles. When all was ready he caused himself to be laid on it, and was carried home.* He was examined by his fellow surgeons and although many wanted to carry out an amputation it was decided to treat it conservatively. He retained his leg and whilst laid up wrote many articles including the management of his fracture (see also Tb page 53).

Treatment

Conservative:

Reduce: Manipulation

Hold: Below knee cast 4-6 weeks

Use: Crutches

Surgical: Fix lateral side with plate and screws, medial, posterior with cancellous screws

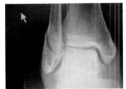 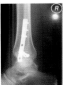 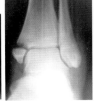 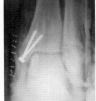

10. FRACTURES OF TALUS/CALCANEUS

Fractures of the neck of the talus may jeopardise the blood supply and accurate reduction necessary

Treatment

Conservative:

> Ice, Elevation, Compression bandage, Crutches, (NonWeightBearing) 2 months

Surgical: Arthrodese subtalar joint if pain persists

11. FRACTURED METATARSALS

a) *Base of 5th*   Common. Crepe bandage, crutches

b) *Neck of 3rd*   (March or stress fracture). Often noted on x-ray with callus present

12. FRACTURED TOES

Aspirate subungual haematoma. Strap to adjacent toe

PERIPHERAL NERVE LESIONS

Nerves are like fibre optic cables that transmit impulses to and from the brain via relay junctions in the spinal cord. They consist of fibres or axons collected into bundles surrounded by a sheath. Damage may be a complete division of a nerve known as a **neurotmesis** or incomplete division with disrupted axons within the sheath called **axonotmesis** or bruising of the nerve called **neuropraxia** where the impulses are unable to be transmitted but the nerve is intact. Following division bleeding occurs at the nerve ends and a clot forms into which grow the axons from the proximal end whilst the distal end degenerates. If the axons are interrupted or obstructed a **neuroma** will form. The growth is usually 1-2mm a day. The distal end of the nerve degenerates and this is known as Wallerian degeneration.

Clinical features depend on the nerve that is damaged, whether it is mixed carrying both motor and sensory fibres or just sensory fibres in which case the area supplied is numb.

Treatment involves repair if there has been division of a nerve which can be **immediate** or **delayed**. If there is a gap between the nerve endings that is too large a nerve graft may be used to provide a nerve graft with an operating microscope and fine materials.

With an axonotmesis or neuropraxia a wait and see approach is adopted.

Multiple nerve injuries such as a brachial plexus lesion in the neck is difficult to treat or a large nerve such as the median or sciatic nerve.

Late treatment may involve tenotomy if muscles are contracted or tendon transfers for example, transferring the tibialis posterior from behind the leg into the tibialis anterior on the front of the leg correcting drop foot deformity.

MUSCLE AND TENDON INJURIES

When a muscle contracts violently it can overcome its tensile strength, producing a tear within the muscle itself or a tear of the tendon.

1.   *ACHILLES TENDON*

A common injury is an Achilles tendon rupture which is felt as a sharp pain above the heel. A gap is palpable in the tendon although the appearance may be normal with the swelling associated. Treatment is usually repair and often the plantaris tendon can be used as a suture material. A cast is applied with the foot in equinus or pointing downwards and is kept in place for 6 weeks. Physiotherapy is necessary afterwards to restore function and strength to the calf.

Conservative treatment can produce a reasonable result but recurrence in more common.

2.   *BICEPS TENDON*

This is commonly in the long head of biceps which passes through the shoulder

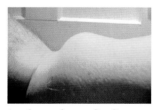 and a characteristic lump appears in the upper arm on stressing the muscle. Pain may be felt prior to this due to inflammation of the tendon known as **tendonitis.** This is the author's right arm. *(There is a spelling mistake which persists in the orthopaedic literature in which inflammation of **tendons** is called **tendinitis**. A book has even been written about it but just because it sounds like it does not mean to say it should be spelt like it and we do not call a below knee plaster a Baloney plaster for example).* Repair is not usually necessary as the other half of the biceps becomes stronger to compensate. It is very common in older men.

83

DISORDERS OF THE UPPER LIMB

1.   *FROZEN SHOULDER (CAPSULITIS)*

This is more common in women usually of middle age producing pain and stiffness and later stiffness and then gradual recovery. The pain is worse at night.

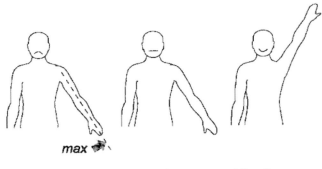

| Initially pain & stiffness | After 1 year stiffness only | After 2 years full recovery |

Treatment: Analgesics and anti-inflammatory tablets

Local injection of steroid

Physiotherapy

Manipulation under anaesthetic (MUA)

It usually resolves slowly over 2 years.

2.   *ROTATOR CUFF LESION*

This may be due to a partial or complete tear of the rotator cuff, usually the supraspinatus tendon. The rotator cuff is a group of muscles attached from the shoulder blade to the upper end of the humerus.   They pass beneath a bony ligamentous arch formed by the articulation between the distal clavicle and the distal spine of the scapula known as the acromion process at the AC or acromioclavicular joint.

There is a painful arc of abduction or inability to lift the arm from the side. The can be due to impingement. Calcification is sometime seen in the tendon as shown in the x-ray.

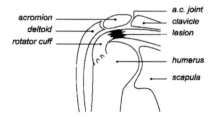 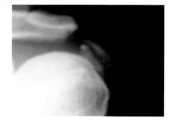

An ultrasound scan or MRI scan can be an aid to diagnosis.

This is the author's right shoulder showing complete rupture with close proximity of the humeral head to the acromion

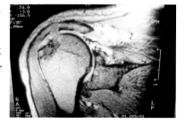

Treatment

Conservative:

a) Analgesics and anti-inflammatories

b) Injection of local anaesthetic and steroid but usually no more than on 3 occasions

c) Physiotherapy in the form of ultrasound. Hydrotherapy, a TENS machine and acupuncture may help.

d) Exercises such as swimming can produce strength in the deltoid to compensate although overhead activities are usually difficult unless surgical intervention takes place.

Surgical:

Surgery is indicated if there has been failure of relief from symptoms by conservative means and where a large tear has been demonstrated by ultrasound scanning. It usually by **arthroscopy and repair,** together with **subacromial decompression,** and often excision of the distal end of the clavicle creating a fibrous arthroplasty at the acromioclavicular joint. Reconstruction is occasionally needed when one can take the latissimus dorsi and transfer this muscle from the humerus to the great tuberosity.

Recovery:

Recovery often takes up to 3 months and physiotherapy is needed to assist.

3. *LATERAL EPICONDYLITIS (Tennis elbow)*

and

4. *MEDIAL EPICONDYLITIS (Golfer's elbow)*

Both are due to an irritation of the extensor and flexor muscle origins, although uncommon in both tennis players and golfers!

Treatment Conservative: Strapping, Topical and systemic anti-inflammatories, Injection LA and steroid, Physiotherapy

Surgical: Release tendon and resuture

5. *REPETITIVE STRAIN INJURY (RSI)*

It is also known as WRULD (work related upper limb disorder). Both are more a descriptive term than a diagnosis. It produces a painful forearm in somewhat emotional young women and often involving compensation and therefore is often not believed but is real to the individual. It is interesting that it is uncommon in pianists or violinists who practice every day.

Treatment: Wrist supports

Change of work environment

6. *DE QUERVAIN'S TENOSYNOVITIS*

This is an inflammation of the extensor tendons at the wrist producing swelling and crepitus. *De Quervain (1868-1940) was a general surgeon in Berne, who was also responsible for the introduction of iodised table salt used in the treatment of goitre.*

Treatment: a)   Topical and systemic anti-inflammatory tablets

b)   Injection of local anaesthetic and steroid

c)   Sometimes release of the tendon sheath

7. *CARPAL TUNNEL*

This is a condition where there is compression of the median nerve at the wrist where it passes through the carpal tunnel together with the tendons that flex the fingers. It is common in middle aged females and affects the thumb, index and middle fingers particularly at night. The patient is often woken up at 2 or 3 o'clock in the morning and shakes the hand. This description is a classic description for the condition. It can be confirmed by nerve conduction studies or EMG.

Treatment

Conservative: Injection of local anaesthetic and steroid and a wrist splint with the hand in extension

Surgical: Release of the flexor retinaculum at the wrist

8.   *TRIGGER FINGER*

This is a condition where there is swelling in the flexor tendon in the palm producing a "catch" or jerk as the finger is bent and straightened. It can be seen in infants with a locked thumb.

Treatment: Percutaneous or open division of the palmar pulley.

9.   *DUPUYTREN'S CONTRACTURE*

This is named after Baron Guillaume Dupuytren (1777-1835), born in poverty who rose to be a leading surgeon in France and Baron of the Empire. It is due to thickening and fibrosis of the palmar fascia in the hand mainly affecting the little and ring fingers which are slowly pulled into the palm.

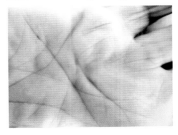 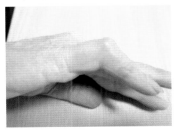

Note the dimples in the palm, and the bent little finger.

Nodules are felt. It can occur in the feet. Excision usually results in cure and if left too late it is difficult to sometimes get the finger out straight again without Z-plasty to the skin and sometimes there is permanent contracture of the MCP (metacarpal phalangeal) or PIP (proximal interphalangeal) joints.

HAND INJURIES

They are important as we are the only animal on the planet able to pick up a pin from the table with our fingers and thumb.

The principles of treatment are to assess the damage, to fix fractures usually internally, to repair vessels and nerves. Elevation and cold packs or ice are used to prevent swelling and it is **most important to maintain and restore function** with exercise as soon as possible.

DISORDERS OF THE KNEE

MENISCAL LESIONS

1. *TEARS*

The menisci in the knee are triangular in cross section and semilunar in shape. The medial meniscus is damaged more commonly than the lateral and in males more than females. It is common in footballers due to planting of the foot and twisting the body with the leg fixed, twisting the knee. The cartilage is split by the overlying femoral condyle and there may be a bucket handle tear or a tear of the anterior or posterior horns.

Symptoms: There is usually a history of a twisting injury

Pain and swelling

Clicking or locking

Sings: A click or clunk on twisting the knee with the knee bent, first described by McMurray

Tests: An x-ray is usually negative but an MRI scan can show a tear

Cross-section of knee

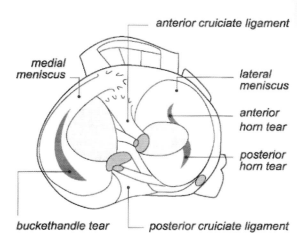

89

Treatment

Conservative: Exercises to strengthen the quadriceps or thigh muscle by swimming and cycling

Physiotherapy

Surgical: Arthroscopic meniscectomy and occasionally repair of peripheral lesions to the capsule. A late complication is arthritis after 20 years or more due to damage to the articular cartilage.

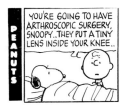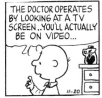

ANTERIOR KNEE PAIN

This is common in young females often due to softening of the lining of the kneecap otherwise called chondromalacia patella.

Treatment:

Conservative   To restrict sporting activities

Physiotherapy

Anti-inflammatory tablets

Surgery: May involve realigning the patellar tendon

Shaving the patella by arthroscopy

Most settle without the need for surgical intervention

CRUCIATE LIGAMENT INJURIES

Rupture of the anterior cruciate (ACL) is common and of the posterior (PCL) uncommon and are often associated with a tear of the medial ligament.

Symptoms: Similar to meniscal lesions with a twisting injury

Signs: a)   There is a positive drawer sign but beware the backward sag of the knee in a PCL tear.

b)   Positive Lachman's test where the leg is grasped firmly and moved relative to the thigh with the knee bent.

c)   A pivot shift test may be positive with a subluxation of the tibia with the knee bent

Tests: a)   MRI

a)   Diagnostic arthroscopy

Treatment
Conservative:

a)   Quadriceps drill

b)   Physiotherapy

c)   Splintage

Surgical:

Repair if acute although mostly late reconstruction is necessary using natural tendons such as the patella or semitendonosis, or synthetic material.   6 months recovery is needed with physiotherapy

SPINAL DISORDERS

The spine consists of a series of **vertebrae** interspersed with **discs** and which moves at the **facet joints**. Movement is effected by the paravertebral muscles which extend from the base of the back to the base of the head. The posterior muscles are stronger than the anterior as the centre of gravity is in front of the spine and they are required to maintain the vertical posture.

Because the spine is angulated at 30° to the horizontal in the lateral plane there is a forward curve in the

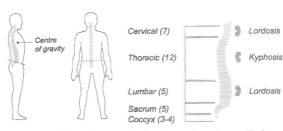

lower back called a **lordosis**, a backward curve in the thoracic spine called a **kyphosis** and a forward curve in the neck called a lordosis to keep the head over the feet. The head is quite heavy weighing 1.5 – 2kg and is supported on a relatively slender column of bone. Most movement occurs in the neck and lower back, as the thoracic spine is relatively stiff to allow the ribs to move. There is very little movement at each individual facet joint and the spine is strengthened by anterior and posterior longitudinal ligaments. There are ligaments between the spinous processes called the interspinous ligaments.

The **disc** is made up of a central nucleus surrounded by an outer laminated annulus fibrosis. It is similar to an old fashioned flattened golf ball which used to be made of a central jelly surrounded by rubber bands and a plastic coat. It gives resilience to the spine. If the annulus becomes worn or if put under abnormal stress the nucleus may bulge through. Pressure

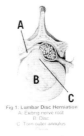

Fig 1: Lumbar Disc Herniation
A: Exiting nerve root
B: Disc
C: Torn outer annulus

on the dura enclosing the **spinal cord** produces **backache** and pressure on the **nerve root** produces **sciatica**.

Most backaches however, are due to stresses and strains in the soft tissues, and are probably due to the fact that we are walking around on two legs on a high gravity planet with a spine that is not properly adapted to the upright posture.

Recovery occurs with exercise, physiotherapy and anti-inflammatory drugs.

Degeneration of the discs is common and commences in the 20s such that by the 60s nearly everybody has some degeneration in the discs whether or not they have symptoms. It is commonly seen at C5/6 and C6/7 and L4/5 and L5/S1.

Coronal view

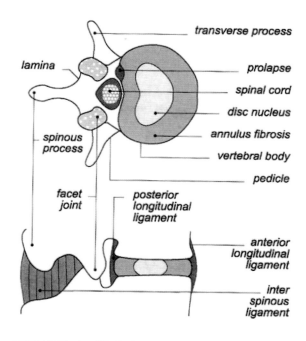

Sagittal view

ACUTE DISC PROLAPSE

This may be due to a blow to the head, sudden movement, heavy lifting or bending. In the neck it produces neck pain and pain radiating down the arm known as **brachialgia** (armatica - author's term) or low back pain and pain radiating down the leg known as **sciatica**.

Signs: Restricted movement

Restricted straight leg raise

Muscle weakness

Altered reflexes

Altered sensation and paraesthesia may occur

This is usually along the dermatomes as shown

Tests: *Plain x-ray* shows loss of lordosis in the neck or back

MRI scan (most helpful). This shows the author's L3/4 disc prolapse with compression of the L4 nerve root and numbness in the dermatome shown and weakness of the quadriceps, with a normal disc for comparison.

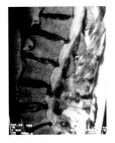
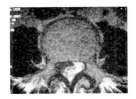
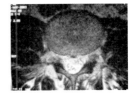

CT scan

Discogram where dye is injected into the disc itself reproducing symptoms

Treatment   Most patients recover without surgery (as did the author, on one occasion (L3/4), requiring surgery on another L5/S1).

Conservative:

> **Rest** (bed rest for 7-10 days) is often helpful with or without traction
>
> **Drugs:Analgesics** such as paracetamol or paracetamol mixed with codeine. I have noticed an increasing tendency for the use of Tramadol which is an opiate analgesic and more likely to produce addiction.
>
> **Anti-inflammatory** tablets provided they do not have side effects upsetting the stomach or provided the patient does not have asthma.
>
> **Antispasmodics** or muscle relaxants such as diazepam or amitriptyline may be helpful in the first 2-3 weeks
>
> **Local splintage** with a collar or corset or brace
>
> The most important is an **exercise programme** such as swimming or cycling and walking without loading the spine
>
> **Physiotherapy**
>
> **Chiropractic**
>
> **Osteopathy**
>
> **Acupuncture**
>
> **Epidural injections**
>
> **Facet joint injections**
>
> **In chronic cases** the use of a pain clinic

Surgical:

Surgical treatment is indicated:

a)   If the patient has bladder symptoms urgent decompression of the spinal cord is necessary, as there may be an underlying cauda equina syndrome

b)   If there has been failure of conservative treatment

c)   There are positive neurological signs

d)   A positive lesion seen on MRI scan

The surgical options are:

a.) Foraminotomy

b) Laminectomy and discectomy with the aid of an operating microscope can be carried out

c) Disc replacement is now used in some situations

d) Spinal fusion if the spine is unstable

CHRONIC/RECURRENT

This is most commonly seen in the low back and is known as the Low Back Syndrome.

Cause: Degenerate discs

Facet joint degeneration

Post traumatic scarring

One should consider alternative pathology such as a rectal carcinoma invading the sacrum or an aortic aneurysm

Symptoms: The pain is usually constant of a deep nagging nature

Radiation if the nerve root is involved

Signs: Reduced movement is noted and in the neck one has to turn the body to reverse the car or use the wing mirrors, and in the low back difficulty in bending to put on socks is often noticed.

Tests: *X-ray*   Reduced disc space is noted with osteophyte formation or lipping

Facet joint narrowing

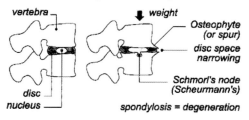

Normal   Degenerative

MRI   Dehydration in the discs, osteophytes, facet joint arthritis.

May show spinal stenosis (narrowing of the canal)

Treatment   The two most important aspects of treatment are:

Weight reduction

Exercise

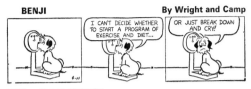

Stopping smoking is important as it has been shown that smoking affects the hydration of the disc with alteration of the vertebral end plate blood flow

A similar regime to the acute disc prolapse is recommended

Surgery: Is indicated if there has been failure of conservative treatment

and may involve:

Decompression

Laminectomy

Spinal fusion

Where compensation is involved there is often a conscious or even an unconscious desire for gain and there are varying distinguishing signs that can be used to recognise patients who are not entirely genuine. Waddell described these some years ago although they were recognised prior to his article.

Signs: Restricted flexion of lumbar spine on standing but normal flexion on sitting up from the lying position

Restricted SLR but can sit up with legs extended (equivalent to SLR 90°). "Cogwheel" flexion of hips with bending knees.

Diminished sensation over the whole limb (glove and stocking) or even the whole side of the body

AMPUTATIONS

Removal of part of the body

Indications:

1. Dead limb – gangrene from arteriosclerosis or severe trauma
2. Lethal limb – may kill patient e.g. severe sepsis, malignant tumour
3. Nuisance – too frail, stiff or deformed

Stump may be:

a) End bearing (weight through end of stump) e.g. through knee amputation. NB scar proximal

b) Non end bearing (weight through soft tissues not end of stump) e.g. below knee amputation. Fish mouth scar

Site of election:

Above knee	(AK) – 11 inches below great trochanter
Below knee	(BK) – 4.5 inches below tibial tubercle
Above elbow	(AE) – 8 inches below tip of acromion
Below elbow	(BE) – 7 inches below tip of olecranon

Technique:

1. Divide muscles, vessels (ligature), nerves (proximal), bone (bevel end)
2. Keep sufficient soft tissue – avoid bony adherence
3. Important to bandage the stump to provide the best stump

Before anaesthesia surgeons had to be very fast especially in the European wars and a surgeon could amputate a leg in a minute. The patients often survived. Remember Long John Silver in" Treasure Island" with his wooden leg or Captain Ahab in "Moby Dick".

4. To fit an artificial limb:

       Immediate pylon

       Delayed fitting

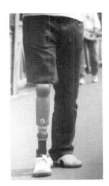

Modern prostheses are very life like.

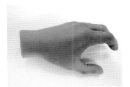 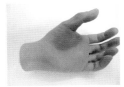 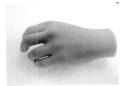

The development of motors may enable some movement.

Below elbow amputation may be treated by separation of radius and ulna to give a pincer (Krukenberg operation)

Complications:

1. Haemorrhage – leave tourniquet on the end of the bed
2. Skin problems with stump (scar too tight) – revise
3. Stump neuroma – excise more proximally
4. Phantom limb – difficult to treat

Definition: Mass of new tissue which persists and grows independently of its surrounding structures. Often called tumours which really only means a swelling.

BENIGN Remains local, suffix *–oma*. Produces symptoms by pressure on surrounding tissue

BONE – Osteoma

    a)   Ivory – lump on skull bones

    b)   Osteoid – central lucent core

            Intense night pain relieved aspirin

            Treat: Excision

    c)   Cancellous – often cartilage capped

CARTILAGE – Chondroma

    a)   Enchondroma inside bone, may cause pathological fracture

    b)   Ecchondroma, outside bone

BONE AND CARTILAGE – Osteochondroma

Bone capped with cartilage – Exostosis

    a)   Single – Usually ends of long bones – points away from growth plate

    b)   Multiple – Diaphyseal aclasis – inherited. 5% become malignant

FIBROUS TISSUE – Fibroma

Fibrous cortical defect. Fibrous dysplasia.

These rarely cause symptoms and show as defects on x-ray with cyst formation or sclerosis

ANEURYSMAL BONE CYST

End of long bones – expansile – symptoms from pressure

UNICAMERAL BONE CYST

Children – ends of long bones (common-humerus).

May present with pathological fracture due to enlarged bone and thin cortex

Treatment for both: Curette and bone graft

HAEMANGIOMA

Rare – spine – backache – striated appearance on x-ray

Treatment: Radiotherapy

INTERMEDIATE

Locally invasive

OSTEOCLASTOMA

Giant cell tumour. Swelling at end of long bone usually in young adults, often painful

Treatment: Curette and bone graft

                Radiotherapy

MALIGNANT

Invade surrounding tissue and metastasise via blood steam and lymphatics to produce secondary deposits

PRIMARY TUMOURS

Rare

OSTEOSARCOMA

Young 10-20, old 5% Paget's disease, often end of long bones. Pain, swelling. Early spread by blood stream.

X-ray: Codman's triangle, sun ray

Treatment: Amputation, radiotherapy, chemotherapy

<50% 5 year survival

CHONDROSARCOMA

Adults flat bones (scapula, pelvis) ends long bone metastasise late

Treatment: Resection

FIBROSARCOMA

Often end femur, proximal tibia. Pain, swelling

Treatment: Amputate

EWING'S TUMOUR

10-20 yrs, mid shaft commonly tibia. Onion skin appearance on x-ray due to new bone formation as periosteum is lifted

Treatment: Excise (amputate) chemotherapy

MULTIPLE MYELOMA

Middle age, pain, x-ray punched out "holes" in bones. Bence-Jones protein in urine

Treatment: Local radiotherapy if practicable

Chemotherapy

LEUKAEMIA

Ache in bones, fatigue (anaemia)

Treatment: Chemotherapy

SECONDARY TUMOURS (METASTASES)

These are the most common form of bone tumours, and although carcinoma spreads mainly via the lymphatics, blood stream spread to multiple sites in bones is common in carcinoma of the:

a)   Breast
b)   Prostate
c)   Lung
d)   Kidney
e)   Thyroid

Bone pain, pathological fractures

Treatment: Internally fix

CARE OF THE DYING PATIENT

1.   Analgesia – do not withhold opiates
2.   Good nursing – soft pillows and sheets, TLC (tender loving care)
3.   Do not resuscitate – death is a release

In this regard there is another story from Paré's war journal: *We entered pell mell into the city and in a stable where we thought to lodge our horses we found four dead soldiers and three propped against the wall. They neither saw, heard nor spoke and their clothes were still smouldering, burned with gunpowder. As I was looking on them with pity, there came an old soldier who asked me if there were any way to cure them: I said, No. Then he went up to them and cut their throats gently and without ill will. I told him he was a villain: he answered he prayed God when he was in such a plight, he might find someone to do the same for him, that he should not linger in misery.*

TUMOURS AND CYSTS OF SOFT TISSUES

Ganglion   Common wrist – jelly

> *Treat:*   Aspirate or excise

Semimembranosus cyst

> Behind knee – common in young boys, trans-illuminates
>
> *Treat:*   Excise

Baker's cyst Behind knee synovial swelling associated arthritis. No treatment

Lipoma   Soft swelling in the subcutaneous tissues, reassure or excise

Fibroma   Firmer lump

Neurofibromatosis

> Multiple lumps in the skin, brown stains (café au lait), giant limbs (elephantiasis)

Neuroma   a) Amputation – pain

Excise more proximally

b) Morton's – Pain, metatarsalgia, sole of foot usually 3-4 cleft between metatarsal heads

Treat: Metatarsal insoles, excise

Bursitis   Inflammatory swelling of bursa over bony prominences

a) Olecranon – drinker's elbow
b) Knee – housemaid's knee (pre-patellar bursitis)

Treat: Anti-inflammatory drugs, injection of local anaesthetic and steroid, excise.

Synovial joints are affected by various disease processes: Rheumatoid arthritis

Osteoarthritis, Gouty arthritis, Anklylosing spondylitis, Hallux rigidus and hallux valgus

RHEUMATOID ARTHRITIS

1. Aetiology: unknown, possibly auto-immune
2. 20-40 female : male 3:1
3. Commences in the synovium: inflamed (synovitis) , thickened (pannus), rheumatoid nodule, effusion
4. Gradually destroys articular cartilage – direct action
5. Ligaments become stretched, lax – deformity
6. Tendon sheaths affected – tendons may rupture (dropped fingers)
7. Relapses and remissions occur – may burn out

Symptoms: Pain, one joint or several (polyarthritis)

Malaise

Stiffness

Signs: Joints swollen, signs of inflammation

Commonly small joints of the hands

Synovial swelling and rheumatoid nodules

Late: deformity Hands – MCP joints – Ulnar drift, dropped fingers (ruptured extensor tendons). IP joints Boutonniere, Swan neck

Feet – Claw toes, bunions and hallux valgus

Tests:	*Blood*	Raised ESR
		Positive Rose Waaler and latex (75%)
		Positive C reactive protein
	X-rays	Osteoporosis, Bone erosion
		Joint space narrowing
		Deformity

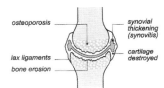

Treatment:

General: Drugs

a)   Analgesics e.g. aspirin (also NSAIDs)

b)   NSAIDs (non steroidal anti-inflammatory drugs) inhibit cyclo-oxygenase (COX) the enzyme producing prostaglandins but also produces side effects such as gastric mucosal irritation

c)   Anti-arthritic, Gold, Chloroquine

d)   Suppressant, Steroids e.g. prednisolone, long term side effects: Cushing's syndrome: thin skin with increased capillary fragility, bruises, osteoporosis, avascular necrosis (hip joint), obesity (moon face, buffalo hump)

e)   TNF – alpha blockers (tumour necrosis factor) e.g. etanercept, infliximab

f)   Methotrexate

Local

a)   Splintage - physiotherapy

b)   Synovectomy

c)   Salvage – arthroplasty

OSTEOARTHRITIS (OA)

Definition: Degeneration in a joint. Degeneration commences in the articular cartilage and can be likened to the wearing out of a carpet. Firstly there is loss of the sheen, then there is gradually loss of the fibre, wear is down to the under-felt and finally through to the floorboards. It is a gradually progressive condition and is common in the weight bearing joints and also the joints of the spine. It is less commonly seen in the upper limb than in the lower limb and surprisingly rare in the ankle although this is the joint most frequently injured by sprains and fractures.

Cause and progression:

1.   Damage to articular cartilage – by trauma, faulty stresses, vascular problems, irritants (e.g. gout) producing chondromalacia – softening and fibrillation of cartilage

2.   Damage to synovial lining – fibrosis of capsule, stretching and pain, gradually restricting movement

3.   Damage to bone:

> Subchondral sclerosis
>
> Osteophyte formation,
>
> lipping
>
> Cysts

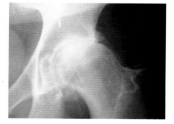

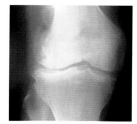

Note the changes in the lateral compartment of the knee, and in the hip.

Symptoms: a)   Pain

          b)   Deformity

          c)   Loss of function

          d)   Limp

          e)   Swelling

Signs: a)   Decreased range of movement

          b)   Crepitus – grating on movement

          c)   Limping – if in joints of the lower limb

          d)   Heberden's nodes in fingers

Tests: *X-ray* a)   Loss of joint space

                 b)   Sclerosis

                 c)   Lipping or osteophyte formation

                 d)   Cysts

Causes of a limp from hip problems throughout life

0-3   DDH

3-5   TB, Transient synovitis (irritable hip)

5-10   Perthe's

0-15   Slipped epiphysis

15-35 Trauma

35-50 OA secondary to preceding conditions

50+   Primary OA

Treatment

General:

a)   Rest – reduce activity, use walking stick

b)   Diet – reduce weight

c)   Drugs: Analgesics, Anti-inflammatories (NSAIDs non-steroidal anti-inflammatory drugs), Glucosamine. Chondroitin, Hyaluronic acid

Conservative:

a)   Heat

b)   Physiotherapy – ultrasound, exercises, shortwave diathermy, massage

c)   Manipulation

d)   Built-up shoe

e)   Injections into joint – Hyaluronate or steroids

f)   Arthroscopy and wash out.

Surgical: Osteotomy, arthroplasty, arthrodesis

<u>**1) Osteotomy**</u> – surgical fracture to alter stresses through joint. Internal or external fixation

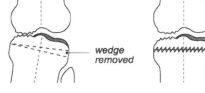

wedge removed

2) **Arthroplasty** – refashion a joint

a) Excision arthroplasty – create a gap to fill with scar tissue by removing part of the bone ends

b) Replace one or both end of the bone with a prosthesis e.g. THR (total hip replacement), TKR (total knee replacement)

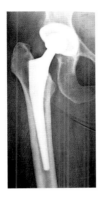 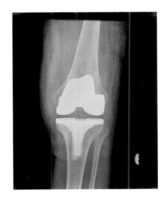

c) Cartilage grafting or possibly stem cell replacement in the future

Complications:

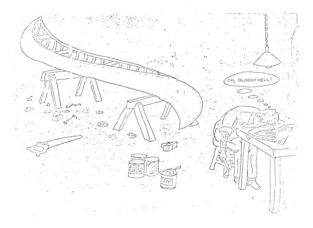

112

General

a) ***Blood loss – shock.*** Treat – blood replacement, may need to re-operate to find bleeding source

b) ***Deep vein thrombosis/pulmonary embolism***

Prevent: Low molecular weight heparin/aspirin, Elastic stockings (TED – thrombo-embolic disease), Calf compression or foot compression pumps in theatre and after surgery

Symptoms: Calf pain, chest pain

Signs: Calf tenderness, pleural rub

Tests: Doppler, Venogram, VQ lung scan

Treatment: Anticoagulants – Heparin 10 days, Warfarin 3 months

Local

a) ***Dislocation***

Prevent: Abduction pillows in hip replacements

Treatment: Relocate – may need to re-operate and change alignment of (usually socket)

b) ***Infection***

Prevent: Preoperative, operative and postoperative broad spectrum antibiotics

Treatment: Antibiotics – Drain. May need exchange prosthesis – difficult. High risk of failure

c)   ***Loosening:*** a late complication usually after 10 years

Prevent: Compression cementing technique, hydroxyapatite coated prostheses in uncemented procedures

Treatment: Revision difficult – operation twice as long as primary procedure. May need to convert to excision arthroplasty (Girdlestone)

3) Arthrodesis

This is fusion of the bone ends. Author's ankle. The trade is loss of pain for loss of movement.

Failure to fuse results in a pseudarthrosis.

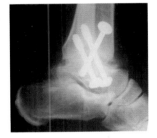

GOUT

This is caused by an increased uric acid level in the blood that produces crystals in the synovium and leads to inflammation. Cartilage may be damaged and lead to arthritis Note the white deposits of uric acid crystals in the knee.

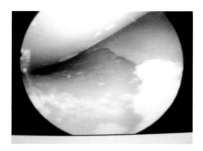

Treatment:

a)   Drugs: Anti-inflammatory; Allopurinol – decreased formation uric acid; Probenecid - increased excretion by kidney

b)   Surgery – as for Osteoarthritis

ANKYLOSING SPONDYLITIS

An inflammatory condition of the spine: progressive, males > females. Commences usually in the sacroiliac joints

Symptoms: Pain, aching more than acute. Stiffness

Signs: Local tenderness

Decreased movement, loss of extension leading to a bent forward position

Tests: *Blood* – HLA antigen positive

X-ray – sclerosis and bone loss in the sacroiliac joints. Bone formation in the apophyseal or facet joints of the spine, ossification of the discs leading to bamboo spine

Treatment

Conservative:

Anti-inflammatory drugs

Physiotherapy – emphasis on exercise and posture

Surgical:

Osteotomy of the spine if the bent forward posture is greater than 45°

HALLUX RIGIDUS : HALLUX VALGUS AND BUNIONS

Hallux rigidus is OA (osteoarthritis) of the metatarsophalangeal (MTP) joint of the big toe and pressure from osteophytes. Treat as for OA

Hallux valgus is an outer sideways deviation of the big toe often associated with a medial or inner deviation of the metatarsal. An exostosis develops on the head of the metatarsal known as a bunion

Symptoms: Pain from pressure of shoes

Signs: Deviated toe, prominent bunion, reduced movement in the MTP joint in hallux rigidus with increased extension in the IP joint. Second toe often too long and forms **hammer toe** with fixed flexion of PIP joint

Tests: *X-rays* show medial deviation of the metatarsal and lateral deviation of the toe with an exostosis (bunion) on the medial side of the 1st metatarsal or osteophytes and joint space narrowing in hallux rigidus.

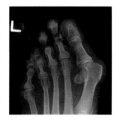

Treatment

Conservative: Relieve pressure by: Felt ring, hole in shoe, metatarsal bar

Surgical:

    a)   Remove bunion – exostectomy

    b)   Osteotomy metatarsal or proximal phalanx

    c)   Arthroplasty : excision (Keller's), replacement (silastic or titanium)

    d)   Arthrodesis – fusion (PIP 2nd toe)

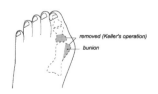

removed (Keller's operation)

bunion

PAGET'S DISEASE

Named after Sir James Paget (1814-1899), one of the great Victorians (it is always interesting to read the biographies of the named scolars and surgeons I have mentioned).

1. Male > female 50-70 age group

2. Cause unknown

Symptoms: Thickening of bone with osteoblastic and clastic activity – spongy soft bone

Signs: Pain, Deformity, Increasing hat size, Bent bones, Stress fractures

Tests: *X-ray* – Mixed osteoporotic and blastic activity

Treatment

Conservative:

Drugs   Analgesics, Fluoride, Biphosphonates

Surgical: Osteotomy

Intramedullary rods for stress fractures in long bone

5% malignant change

VITAMIN DEFICIENCY

Vitamin D   Rickets – soft bones especially distal tibia. Prevent by exposure to sunlight to stimulate melanoblasts and treat with vitamin supplement.

Vitamin C   Scurvy – subperiosteal haemorrhage

Pain, loose teeth

Treat: Fresh fruit, Vitamin supplement

(British sailors in the 18th Century were known as Limeys as they were provided with limes to prevent scurvy on long voyages)

OSTEOMALACIA

Loss of calcium from bone – malnutrition, post gastrectomy.

Treat: Calcium, vitamin D

OSTEOPOROSIS

Loss of calcium as absorption greater than formation leads to decreased quantity of bone

1. Postmenopausal
2. Disuse
3. Elderly
4. Dowager hump

Pathological fractures common

Treatment: HRT (hormone replacement therapy, Exercises (most important), Treat fractures as appropriate. No response to vitamin D but use of Calcichew and Alendronate.

COMPLEX REGIONAL PAIN SYNDROME

Previously called Reflex Sympathetic Dystrophy

This is an altered vascular response, often to minor trauma and leads to demineralisation of bone, changes in the skin and disabling pain which is difficult to treat. Spontaneous resolution can occur. Sympathectomy in some cases.

FIBROMYALGIA

Chronic pain syndrome but diagnosis still somewhat in dispute

Everyone has problems and sometimes people find relief from their problems through imaginary illness, or gaining attention from real illness. The glass seems to be half empty rather than half full.

Placebo medication (no active ingredients) can provide relief in about 30% of cases, even with known diseases.

Where a true psychotic state exists a diagnosis of conversion hysteria can be made. Treatment is extremely difficult.

The system of payment for injury may result in patients not wanting to get better from genuine injuries or feigning symptoms and signs (malingering), and the examining doctor for the Court has to be as objective as possible. The system of blame and claim seems to becoming more and more prevalent, fuelled by lawyers. "I have been hurt and someone must pay for my pain and loss of amenity" is a common underlying, though often not able to be expressed, thought process. It is similar in divorce where revenge is taken on the partner, (usually the husband), for the breakdown of the marriage through obstruction to access where there are children.

With children, abuse must be suspected if a fracture occurs under the age of two with a doubtful history, and there are numerous examples of a child being returned to abusive parenets because doctors, nurses and social workers do not suspect that some parents could mistreat their children.

We all have our own foibles and must be as objective and understanding as possible when dealing with patients.

Doctors are in a position where they can help many people return to health and most doctors enter the profession to do just that.

However, sometimes mistakes happen e.g. prescribing a drug where there is a known allergy, or an injection wrongly sited damaging a nerve for example. There is no guarantee in medicine but an expectation that treatment will be successful.

Negligence is accepted where a doctor falls **below** the standard of care considered by his peers to be reasonable. Often it is the system at fault and not just the individual and when deficiencies in practice occur the whole approach must be examined.

When administering a drug or giving a blood transfusion it is always best to check the dose or blood label with a second person. Giving adult doses to children is a common mistake, or mistaking milligrams for micrograms.

A doctor or patient should never be embarrassed about getting a second opinion, particularly if major surgery is involved.

Advice must be tempered with knowledge and it is important to have a clear understanding of what treatment is to be given, before undertaking that treatment, and making sure consent is given on the basis of understanding.

As one teacher said to me "Know thy limitations" and I pass it on to you.

Summary

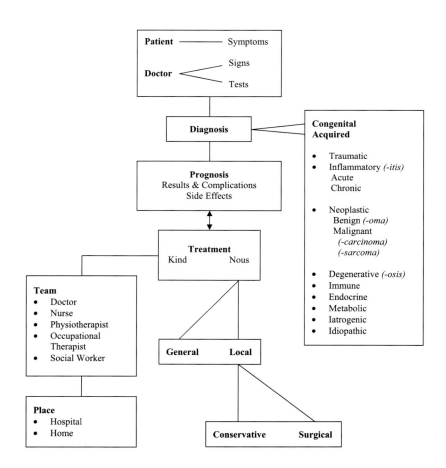

INDEX

A

Abduction 24
Abscess 17
Accident – major 64
Acetabulum-
    CDH/DDH 34
    Fracture 78
Achilles tendon rupture 83
Achondroplasia 42
Acromioclavicular joint 65,85
Acquired 17
Acromegaly 21
Acupuncture 69
Adduction 24
Adolescent kyphosis 44
Airway 64
Alimentary system 10
Amputation 99
Andry, Nicholas 5
Aneurysmal bone cyst 103
Ankle 12, 79
Ankylosing spondylitis 117
Annulus fibrosis 92,93
Anterior 25
Anterior cruciate ligament 89,90
Anterior knee pain 91
Apley, Alan Graham 2
Apophysis 15
Apophysitis -
    Osgood Schlatter's 45
    Sever's 45
Arteriography 27
Arthritis 20,
    Degenerative 109
    Gout 115
    Infective (septic) 51
    Osteo 109
    Rheumatoid 107
Arthrodesis 29,114
Arthroplasty 29, 112
Arthroscopy 29,86, 89,90
Arthrotomy 29
Articular cartilage 13,109
Athetosis 42
ATLS 64
Atlas 13
Atom 6

Avascular necrosis 61,76
Avulsion fractures 67, 74
    Axon 9
    Axontmesis 82

B

Back ache/pain 20, 93
Baker's cyst 105
Benign tumours 19, 101
Biceps tendon rupture 83
Bicipital tendonitis 83
Blood supply of bone 14
Bone - Cancellous 14
    Compact 14
    Scan 27
Bone graft 61
Bone growth 15
Bone mineral density 27
Bow leg 40
Brachialgia 68,94
Brittle bone 43
Bursa, bursitis 106

C

Calcaneus 12, 81
Calcaneo-valgus 39
Calcification 15, 58, 85
Calcium 14, 120
Calcium hydroxyapatite 14
Capsule 13, 54,
Capsulitis 84
Cardio-vascular system 9
Care of dying 104
Carpal 12
Carpal tunnel 87
Cartilage 13, 89, 101
CDH 34
Cells 9, 11
Cerebral palsy 42
Cervical spine25, 68
Cervical spondylosis 20,73,93
Chondroma 19,101
Chondromalacia patella 90,109
Chondrosarcoma 103
Clavicle 12,64
Club foot 38
Coccydnia 74

Haemo-poietic system 10
Hallux rigidus, valgus 117
Hammer toe 117
Hand injuries 88
Harness 36
Harris line 35
Healing of fracture 58
Heberden's nodes 110
Heel fractures calcaneus 81
Hemiplegia 72
Hip -
        Fractures 75
        Dislocation 77
Humerus 12, 64
Hydrogen 6
Hypertrophy 15

I

Iatrogenic 21, 122
Idiopathic 21
Ilium 12
Infection 48
Inferior 24
Inflammation 17
Intervertebral disc 92,93
Intoeing 40
Ischium 12
-itis 17

J
Joint 13

K
Keller's117
Knee –
        Joint 12
        Fractures 78
        meniscal lesions 89
Knock knee 40
Kyphosis 47, 92
Kyphus 70

L
Lamina 93
Laminectomy 96
Lateral 24

Leg -
        Bow 40
        Fractures 79
Leukaemia
Ligament 13,78
Limp 110
Loose bodies 45
Lordosis 47,92
Lower limb fractures 75
Lumbar spine 92
Lunate 66
Lymphatic system 10
- lysis 29

M
Magnetic Resonance Imaging 26
Malignant tumours 19
Mallet finger 66
Mal-union 61
Mandible 12
March fracture 81
Medial 24
Meningo-myelocoele 41
Meniscus 13
Meniscal tears 89
Mesoderm 8
Metacarpal 12
        fractures 66
Metaphysis 15
Metastasis 19,104
Metatarsal 12
        Fracture 81
MRI 26,85,94
Morton's neuroma 106
Munchausen's syndrome 21
Muscles- 16
        cardiac, smooth, striated 16
Muscle strength 52
Myeloma 104

N
Neck – femur fractures 75
Negligence 122
Neoplastic 19
Nerve lesions 82
Nervous system 9